CONTENTS

Why eat vegetables?
Make half your plate vegetables and fruits
Shopping tips
Food safety
Vegetable guide
Recipes
    Step-by-step: Steaming
    Step-by-step: Roasting
    How much do I need for a recipe?
    Breakfasts
    Soups
    Salads
    Sides
    Salsas, sauces and dips
    Main dishes

I ♥ VEGETABLES
Choosing, Cooking, Eating and Enjoying More Vegetables

1st edition, Copyright 2018, Fresh Baby LLC

All rights reserved. This book, or parts thereof, may not be reproduced in any form without permission.

Published by Fresh Baby LLC

523 East Mitchell Street, Petoskey, MI 49770

www.freshbaby.com

ISBN: 978-0-9895938-0-9

Author: Cheryl Tallman

Cover and Book Design: Dylan Tallman, Creative i

Food Photography: Roger Tallman, Creative i

Printed in Korea

Why eat vegetables?

Eating vegetables every day is a great way to feel better and live longer. Vegetables are one of the five main food groups. It is difficult to find another food group that is as perfectly matched to our everyday health as vegetables. Vegetables are **low in calories** and high in fiber. This means that you can eat a large portion of them and feel full (thanks to the fiber).

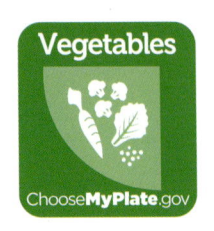

As a group, vegetables are **excellent sources of many essential vitamins and minerals**. The body cannot make vitamins, so we have to get them from the foods we eat. Eating vegetables every day provides your body with a supply of important vitamins.

In addition to vitamins and minerals, vegetables **have a lot of phytonutrients**. In the science of food, phytonutrients are linked to prevention of certain diseases and decreasing risks of certain cancers.

Vegetables also provide **amazing digestive benefits** that come from their high-fiber content. Getting enough dietary fiber is critical for good health; including fiber in all meals and snacks ensures that food moves through our digestive system in a healthy way. The great news is that vegetables are some of the richest sources of fiber that exist.

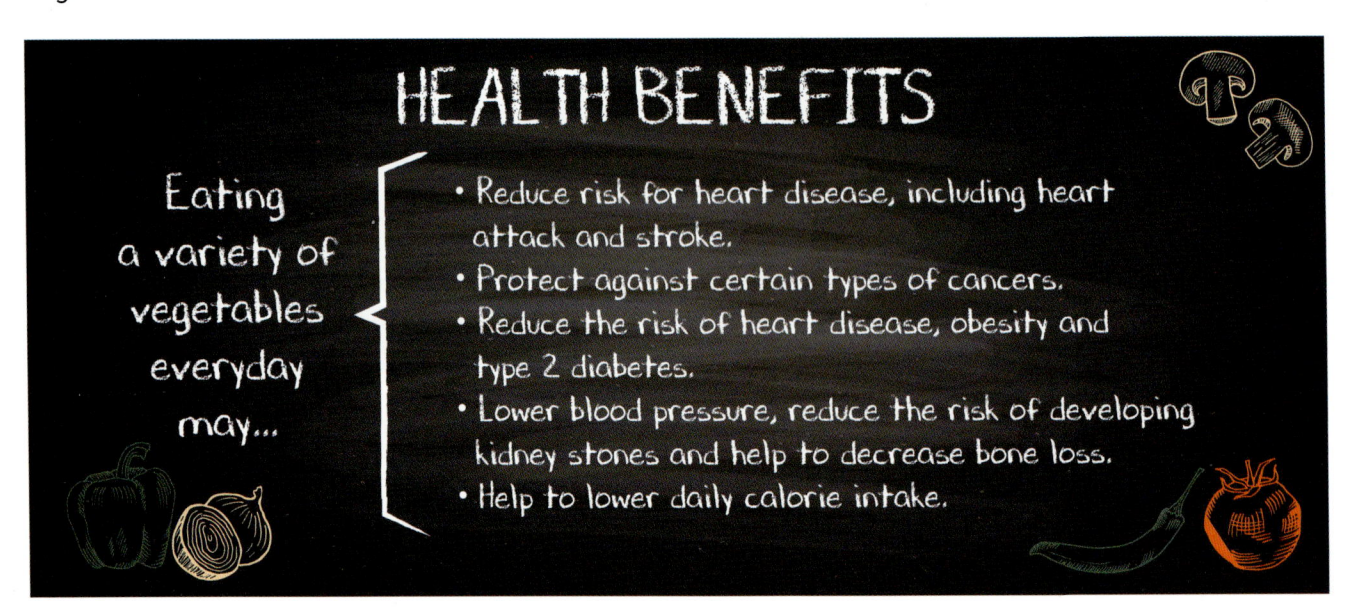

HEALTH BENEFITS

Eating a variety of vegetables everyday may...

- Reduce risk for heart disease, including heart attack and stroke.
- Protect against certain types of cancers.
- Reduce the risk of heart disease, obesity and type 2 diabetes.
- Lower blood pressure, reduce the risk of developing kidney stones and help to decrease bone loss.
- Help to lower daily calorie intake.

Vary your veggies

Any vegetable or 100% vegetable juice counts as a member of the vegetable group. Vegetables can be raw or cooked; fresh, frozen, canned, or dried; and may be whole, cut-up, or mashed.

The vegetable food group is divided into five groups. Each group of vegetables provides the body with different vitamins, minerals and phytonutrients. Eating a variety of vegetables from these five groups helps to make sure that your body gets the nutrients it needs.

Vegetable groups

Dark green
- Broccoli
- Spinach
- Collard greens

Red & orange
- Carrot
- Sweet potato
- Acorn squash

Legumes
- Black beans
- Chickpeas
- Lentils

Starchy
- Corn
- Peas
- Potato

Other
- Cabbage
- Cauliflower
- Celery

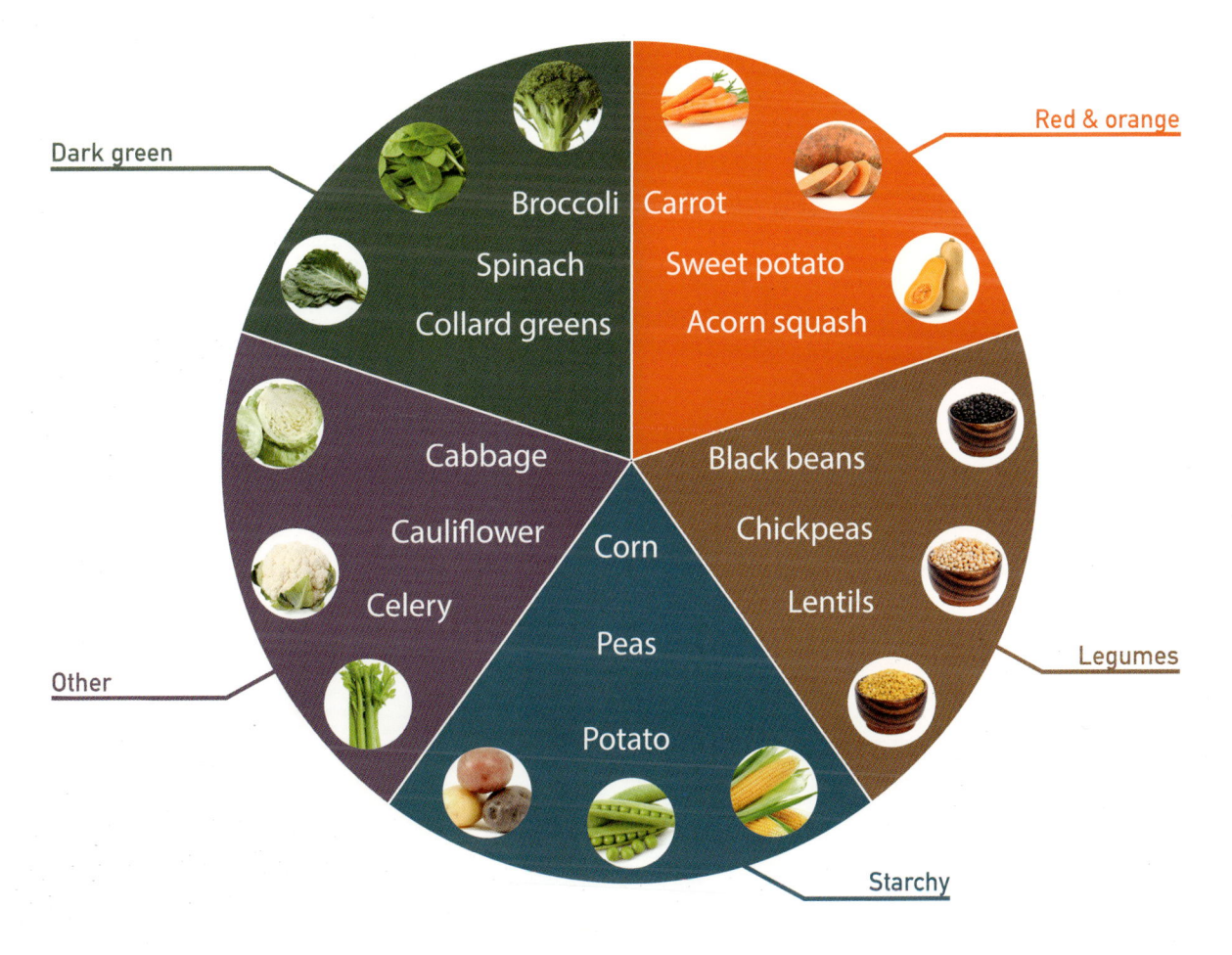

3

Make half your plate vegetables and fruits

The U.S. Dietary Guidelines recommended daily amount of vegetables depends on your age, gender and level of physical activity.

Daily Vegetable Guide*	
Children	
2-3 years old	1 cup
4-8 years old	1 ½ cups
Girls	
9-13 years old	2 cups
14-18 years old	2 ½ cups
Boys	
9-13 years old	2 ½ cups
14-18 years old	3 cups
Women	
19-30 years old	2 ½ cups
31-50 years old	2 ½ cups
51+ years old	2 cups
Men	
19-30 years old	3 cups
31-50 years old	3 cups
51+ years old	2 ½ cups

* These amounts are appropriate for individuals who get less than 30 minutes per day of moderate physical activity, beyond normal daily activities. Those who are more physically active may be able to consume more while staying within calorie needs.
Source: USDA Center for Nutrition Policy and Promotion, Choosemyplate.gov

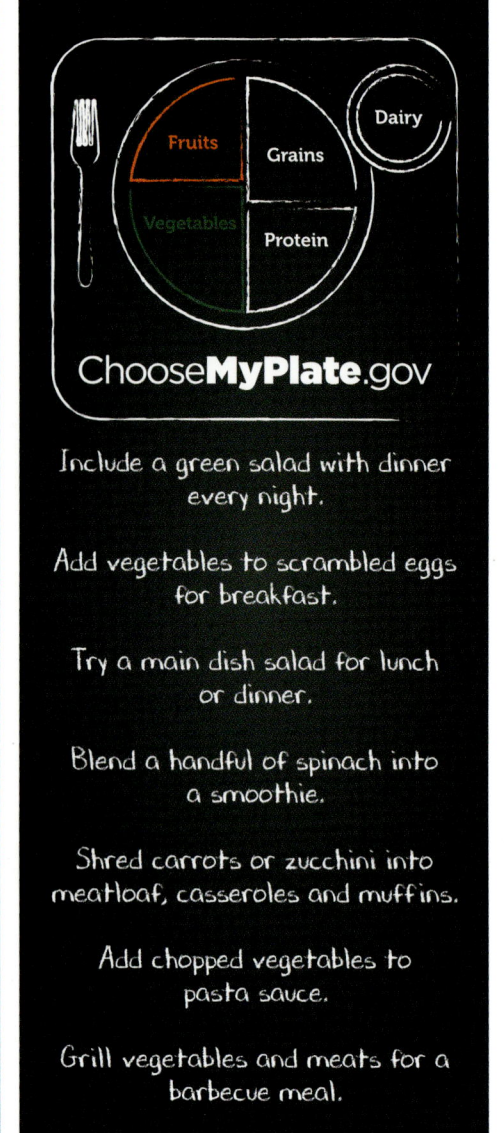

ChooseMyPlate.gov

Include a green salad with dinner every night.

Add vegetables to scrambled eggs for breakfast.

Try a main dish salad for lunch or dinner.

Blend a handful of spinach into a smoothie.

Shred carrots or zucchini into meatloaf, casseroles and muffins.

Add chopped vegetables to pasta sauce.

Grill vegetables and meats for a barbecue meal.

How much is a 1 cup serving?

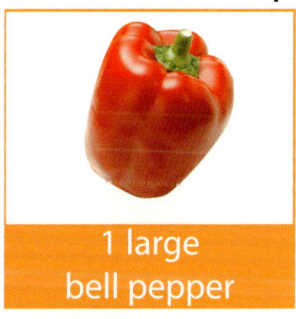

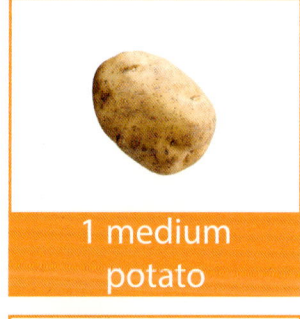

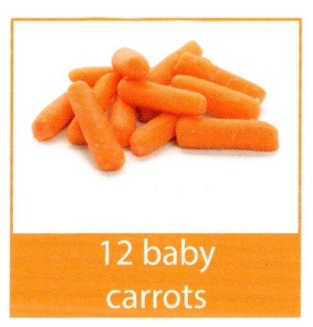

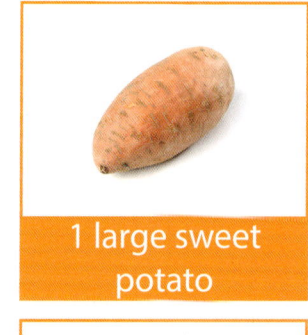

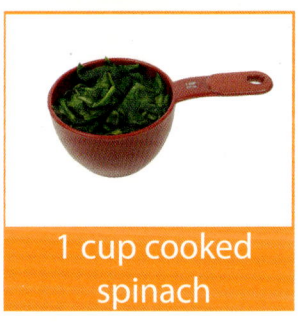

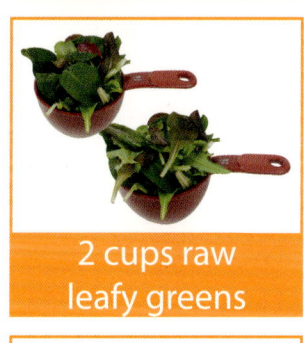

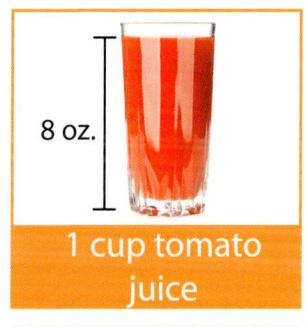

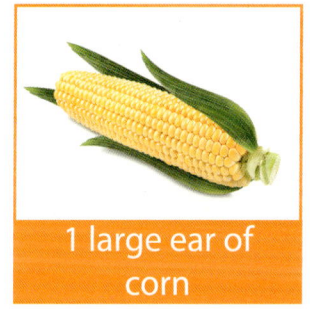

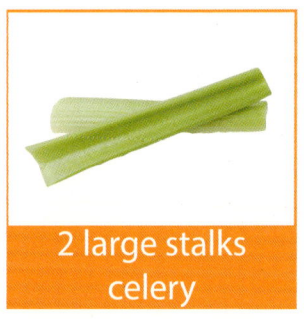

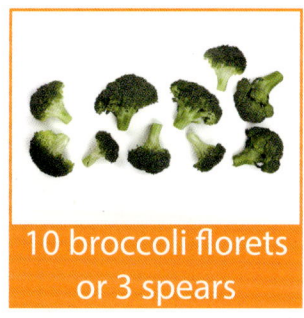

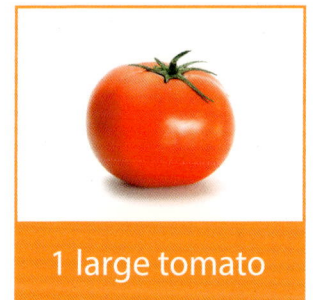

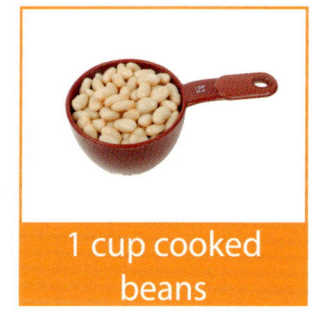

1 large bell pepper	1 medium potato
12 baby carrots	1 large sweet potato
1 cup cooked spinach	2 cups raw leafy greens
1 cup tomato juice (8 oz.)	1 large ear of corn
2 large stalks celery	10 broccoli florets or 3 spears
1 large tomato	1 cup cooked beans

Visual Guide for Portion Sizes

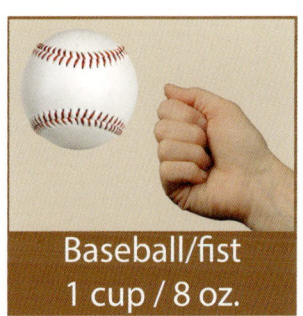

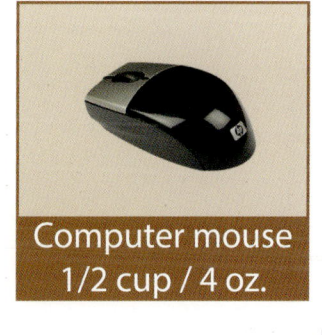

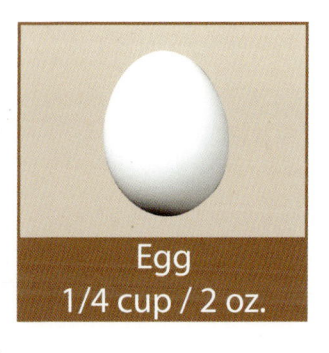

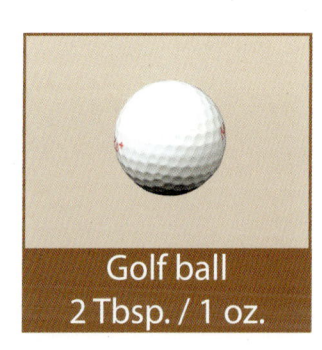

Baseball/fist — 1 cup / 8 oz.	Computer mouse — 1/2 cup / 4 oz.
Egg — 1/4 cup / 2 oz.	Golf ball — 2 Tbsp. / 1 oz.

Tips for shopping for fresh vegetables

- **Buy vegetables on sale:** An item on sale sells faster than a non-sale item. Faster moving foods get restocked more regularly, making them fresher.
- **Buy in season:** Vegetables that are "in season" are fresh, flavorful and often on sale.
- **Buy locally grown:** Locally grown produce is usually fresher and supports farmers in your community. You can buy local produce at a farmers market, or look for grocery store signs that indicate the item was grown near you!
- **Use your senses:** Smell it, look at it and feel it to check for freshness. Not all vegetables have a particular smell, but they should not smell moldy or rotten. Skin colors should be bright; not shriveled or have soft spots or bruises. Packaged vegetables should be free of mold and liquids.
- **Check the expiration date on packages:** Make sure your vegetables are not past this date.
- **Weigh your options:** Compare prices, some prepackaged fruits and vegetables with a fixed price may be cheaper than the same item priced individually or by the pound.

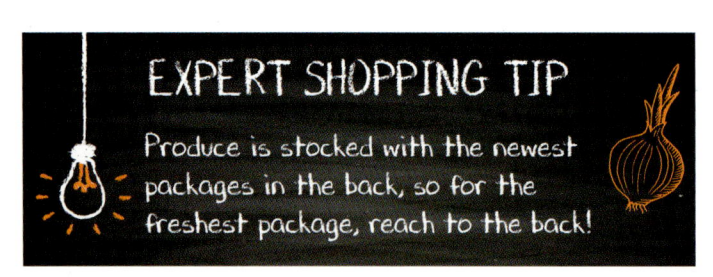

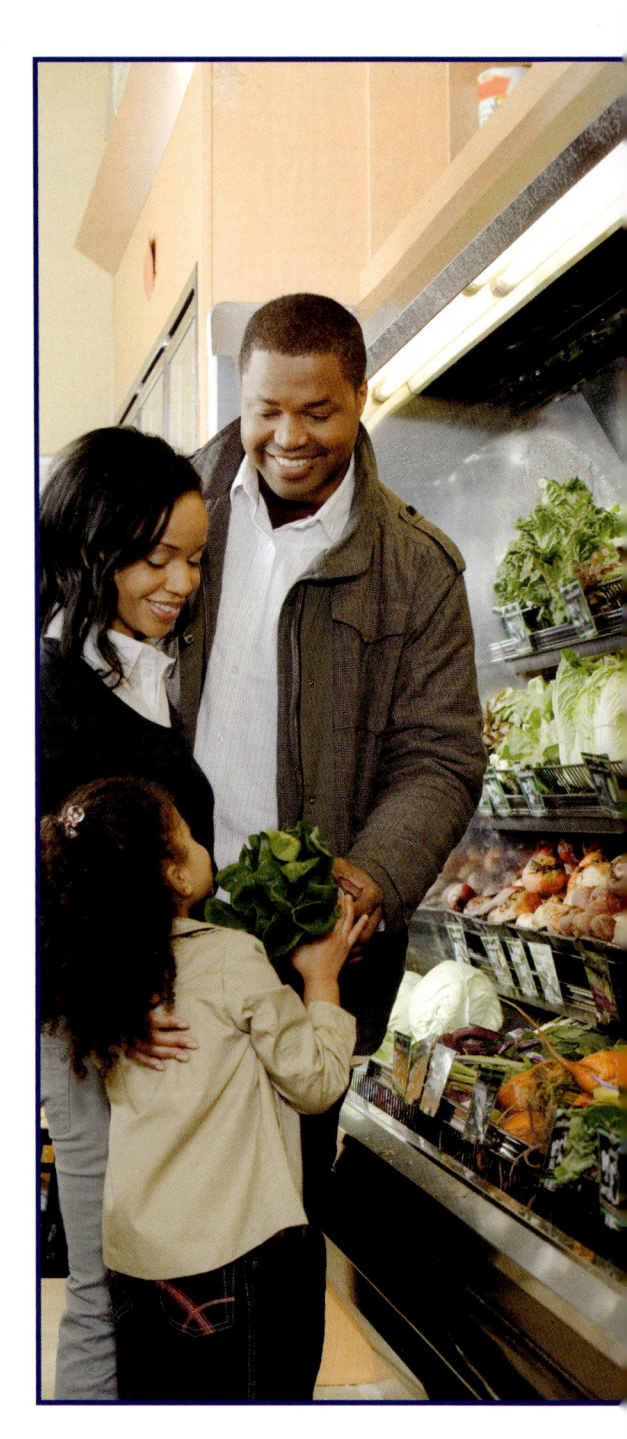

EXPERT SHOPPING TIP

Produce is stocked with the newest packages in the back, so for the freshest package, reach to the back!

Making the most of a farmers market

Shopping at a farmers market is the easiest way to eat fresh, locally grown food and support the farmers in your community, plus it's a fun way to get grocery shopping done! A farmers market is a great place to learn about new foods too. If you see an unfamiliar food, ask about it, farmers are very helpful.

Here are some questions that can help you learn more about a new vegetable and how to enjoy it:
- What does this vegetable taste like?
- Do I eat it this raw?
- What is the best way to cook this?
- Is this ready to eat today?
- How can you tell if this is ripe?

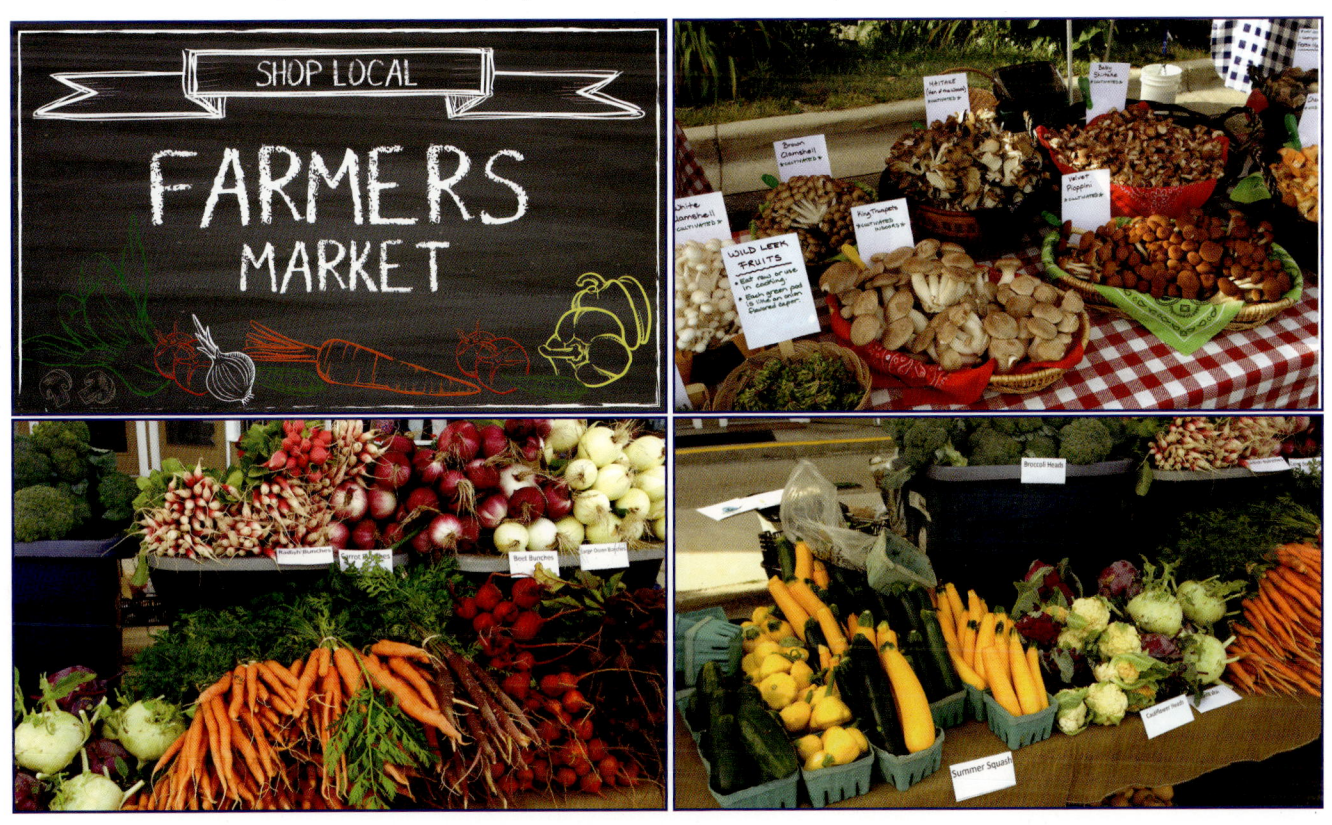

Canned, frozen and dried vegetables

When it comes to making healthy food choices, all forms of fruits and vegetables count toward your daily recommendation including fresh, frozen, canned and dried.

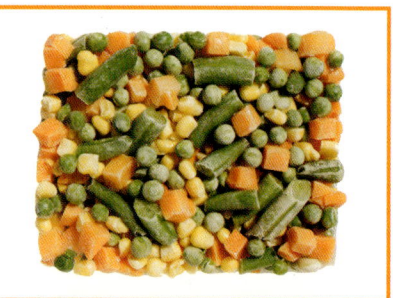

Did you know?
- Frozen vegetables require little preparation. For instance, washing and slicing are already done, saving you time!
- When buying frozen pre-seasoned vegetables, check the nutrition facts label for the amounts of sodium and fat. It is healthier and cheaper to buy the unseasoned frozen vegetables and add your own seasonings at home.
- Canned foods are "cooked" prior to packaging, so they are ready to eat as soon as they are opened.
- Buy canned vegetables labeled "reduced sodium," "low sodium," or "no salt added" so that you can control the salt content.
- Dried vegetables last longer than fresh vegetables.
- Dried vegetables are great added to soups and stews, where the liquid helps restore the original consistency.

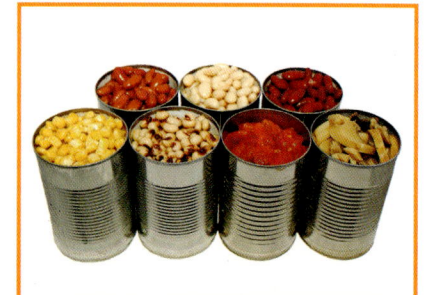

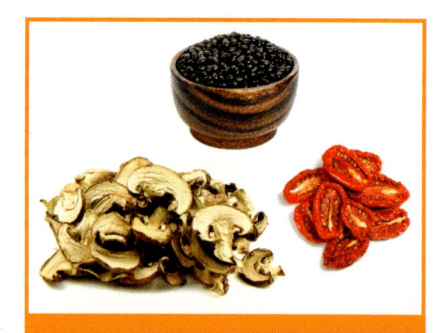

Frozen vegetables

Canned vegetables

Dried vegetables

KEEP IT SAFE AND CLEAN IN THE KITCHEN!

Wash your hands for at least 20 seconds with soap and warm water before preparing or eating food.

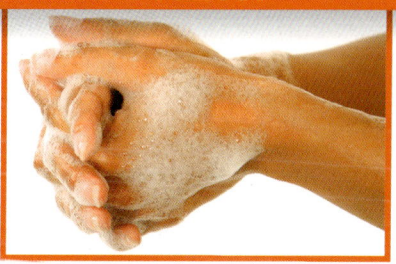

PREVENT CROSS CONTAMINATION

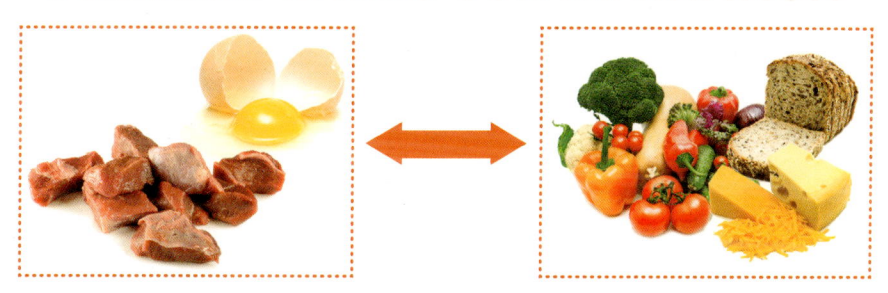

Keep raw meat, poultry, fish and their juices away from other food. After cutting raw meats, wash hands, cutting board, knife and counter tops with hot, soapy water.

STORING FRUITS + VEGETABLES

- Promptly store produce that needs refrigeration.
- Fresh, whole produce such as bananas and potatoes don't need refrigeration.
- Refrigerate all produce that is purchased pre-cut, bagged or peeled.
- Refrigerate fresh produce within two hours of peeling or cutting.
- Throw away cut produce left at room temperature for more than two hours.

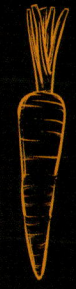

PREPARATION

Wash fruits and vegetables under running water just before eating, cutting or cooking.

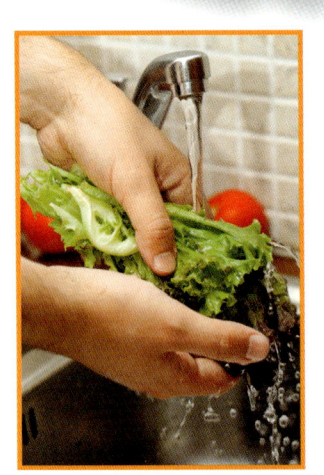

- Some vegetables, such as potatoes, cucumbers and carrots can be scrubbed with a produce brush.
- Cut away and throw out bruised or damaged areas of fruits and vegetables.
- Remove and throw out outer leaves of lettuce.
- Use clean scissors or blades to open bags of produce.
- If a fruit or vegetable looks rotten, throw it out.

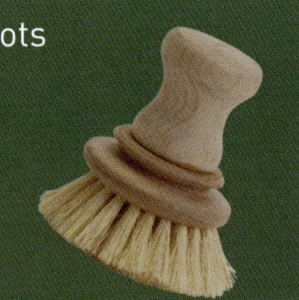

Keep hot food hot and cold food cold!

**Never leave food out over 2 hours.
(or 1 hour in temperatures above 90°F)**

Welcome to the veggie guide!

The next few pages will introduce a wide variety of vegetables that are commonly available in grocery stores and local farmers markets throughout the United States. This easy-to-follow guide offers support for choosing, storing, prepping and eating vegetables.

Using the veggie guide

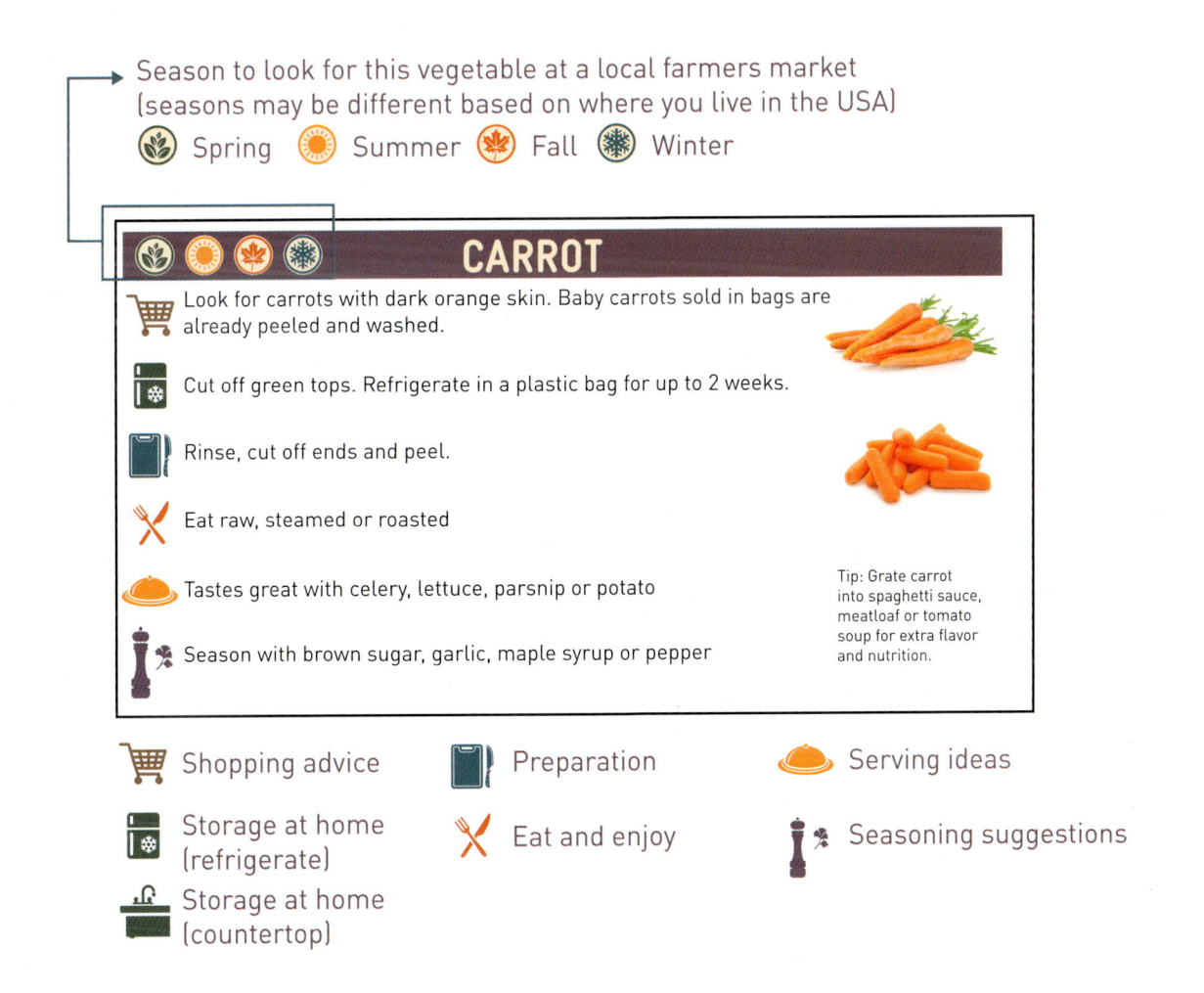

Season to look for this vegetable at a local farmers market (seasons may be different based on where you live in the USA)

Spring   Summer   Fall   Winter

CARROT

- Look for carrots with dark orange skin. Baby carrots sold in bags are already peeled and washed.
- Cut off green tops. Refrigerate in a plastic bag for up to 2 weeks.
- Rinse, cut off ends and peel.
- Eat raw, steamed or roasted
- Tastes great with celery, lettuce, parsnip or potato
- Season with brown sugar, garlic, maple syrup or pepper

Tip: Grate carrot into spaghetti sauce, meatloaf or tomato soup for extra flavor and nutrition.

- Shopping advice
- Storage at home (refrigerate)
- Storage at home (countertop)
- Preparation
- Eat and enjoy
- Serving ideas
- Seasoning suggestions

11

ASPARAGUS

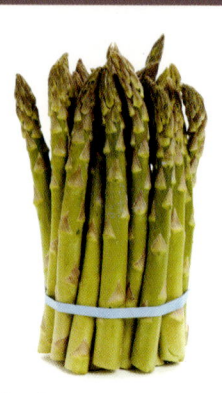

- 🛒 Choose bright green, firm, straight stalks with compact tips. Avoid limp and wilted stalks.
- 🧊 Wrap the ends of the stalks with damp paper towel and store in a plastic bag. Refrigerate for up to 5 days.
- 🔪 Rinse and snap off ends.
- 🍴 Eat raw, blanched, steamed, sautéed, roasted or grilled
- 🍽️ Tastes great with parmesan cheese, egg, soy sauce, green onions, mushrooms or tomato
- 🧂 Season with pepper, lemon or ginger

Tip: Steam asparagus, toss with olive oil and lemon pepper. Sprinkle with parmesan cheese. Serve.

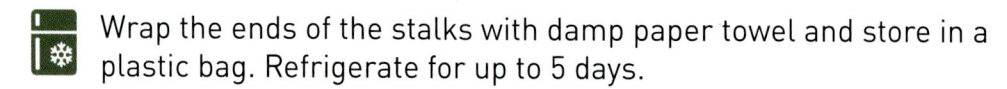

AVOCADO

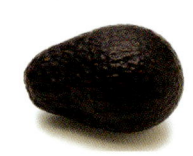

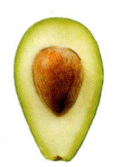

- 🛒 Choose an avocado that is heavy for its size, not too hard and without dark or soft spots.
- 🧊 To ripen, store on the countertop or in a paper bag. For ripe avocados, refrigerate up to 3 days.
- 🔪 Cut avocado in half longwise with a sharp knife. Separate the two pieces by twisting them in opposite directions. Remove the pit with a spoon. Peel off skin, then slice or dice into pieces.
- 🍴 Eat raw
- 🍽️ Tastes great with black beans, chicken, mango, sour cream or tomato
- 🧂 Season with cilantro, lemon, lime or salad dressing

Tip: Avocados brown quickly, prep them just before eating and sprinkle with lemon or lime juice to slow down any browning.

BEETS

- Choose smaller-sized, smooth skinned, dark red or yellow beets with firm roots.

- Cut the greens off beets and refrigerate in a plastic bag for up to 3 weeks.

- To eat raw: Rinse, peel, then grate or slice raw beets to use in salads. To eat cooked: Rinse, then remove the skin after they are cooked.

- Eat raw, steamed or roasted

- Tastes great with carrots, creamy salad dressing, hard-boiled egg or onion

- Season with cinnamon, cumin, dill or tarragon

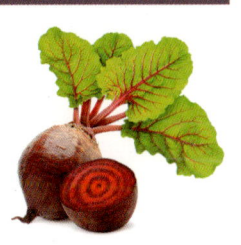

Tip: When adding beets to a salad, toss them first with salad dressing then add to the salad just before serving. This will prevent the beets from turning the whole salad purple.

BELL PEPPERS

- Choose peppers that feel heavy for their size, with glossy skin and no soft spots.

- Refrigerate unwashed for up to 5 days.

- Rinse, then cut in half, remove stem, core, white part and seeds. Alternatively, cut all four sides off and throw away the core.

- Eat raw, stir-fried, roasted or grilled

- Tastes great with pasta, potato, onion, rice or tomato

- Season with basil, garlic, lemon or oregano

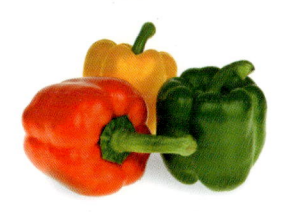

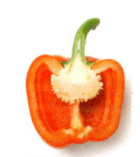

Tip: Different colored peppers have different flavors; green is slightly bitter and red, orange or yellow are sweet.

BROCCOLI

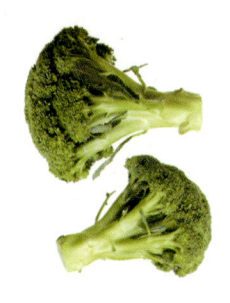

🛒 Look for light green stalks and bright green or purplish-green heads. Don't buy broccoli with yellow heads.

🧊 Refrigerate unwashed for up to 5 days.

🧼 Wash before using. Remove any leaves. Both stems and flowers can be eaten.

🍴 Eat raw, blanched, steamed, stir-fried or roasted

🍽 Tastes great with breadcrumbs, cauliflower, cheese or chicken

🧂 Season with curry, garlic or lemon

Tip: Lemon juice is an easy, flavorful seasoning for broccoli. Add the juice right before serving to avoid the broccoli turning gray-green color.

BRUSSELS SPROUTS

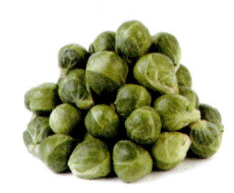

🛒 Look for a selection with a bright green coloring. Yellow spots indicate rotting.

🧊 Refrigerate unwashed in a plastic bag for up to 1 week.

🧼 Rinse. Slice off the base end and remove outside leaves.

🍴 Eat raw, steamed, stir-fried or roasted

🍽 Tastes great with carrot, cauliflower, mushrooms or potato

🧂 Season with basil, garlic, rosemary or thyme

Tip: Brussels sprouts are done if you can poke them easily with a fork. Smaller ones cook faster than larger ones.

CABBAGE

- Choose firm heads with shiny, loose outer leaves.
- Refrigerate for up to 1 week.
- Remove the outer leaves and run it under cold water. Cut the cabbage into quarters, then cut the hard-white core out of each piece.
- Eat raw, stir-fried or roasted
- Tastes great with apple, bacon, carrot, onion or potato
- Season with caraway seed, honey, lemon or thyme

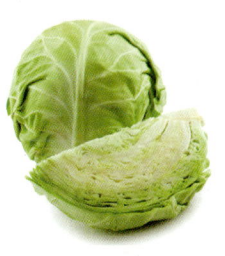

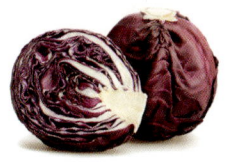

Varieties: Red, Green, Savoy, Napa and Bok Choy

CARROT

- Look for carrots with dark orange skin. Baby carrots sold in bags are already peeled and washed.
- Cut off green tops. Refrigerate in a plastic bag for up to 2 weeks.
- Rinse, cut off ends and peel.
- Eat raw, steamed or roasted
- Tastes great with celery, lettuce, parsnip or potato
- Season with brown sugar, garlic, maple syrup or pepper

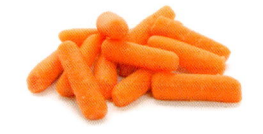

Tip: Grate carrot into spaghetti sauce, meatloaf or tomato soup for extra flavor and nutrition.

CAULIFLOWER

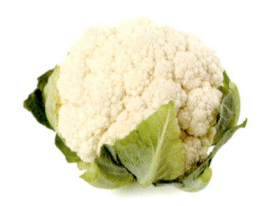

- Look for cauliflower that is firm with a creamy white color. The leaves should be crisp and a bright green.
- Refrigerate in a plastic bag for up to 5 days.
- Remove the outer leaves. Separate the white florets from the head by cutting them off the stalk. Rinse florets.
- Eat raw, blanched, steamed or roasted
- Tastes great with asparagus, beef, broccoli, peas or sweet potato
- Season with chives, curry powder, dill or garlic

Tip: Finely chopped cauliflower is a tasty substitute for rice. Simply sauté it in olive oil until tender, season with salt and pepper and serve.

CELERY

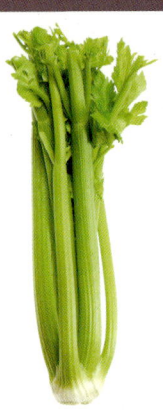

- Choose firm, shiny stalks without yellow or brown leaves.
- Refrigerate in a plastic bag for 1 week or more.
- Cut off base and leaves, separate the stalks and rinse. The tougher strings can be removed with a peeler.
- Eat raw or stir-fried
- Tastes great with apple, barley, carrot, cream cheese, peanut butter or raisins
- Season with dill, parsley or tarragon

Tip: Stuff celery with cheese, tuna, egg salad or peanut butter for a simple snack.

COLLARD GREENS

- 🛒 Choose firm, crisp and deep green leaves with no yellowing or browning.
- ❄️ Refrigerate in a plastic bag for up to 5 days.
- 🔪 Rinse, remove thick stems and chop.
- 🍴 Eat steamed or stir-fried
- 🍽️ Tastes great with black-eyed peas, brown rice, potato or quinoa
- 🧂 Season with garlic, lemon or pepper

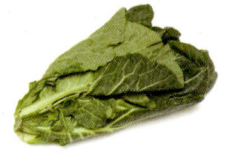

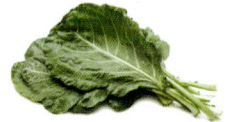

CORN

- 🛒 Choose husks that are bright green with moist yellow/brown tassels. Pull back the husk at the top, the kernels should be plump.
- ❄️ Refrigerate with the husk on. Remove husk just before cooking. Eat within 2 days of purchase.
- 🔪 Remove husk, remove the silk and snap off stalk. For grilling, leave the husks on.
- 🍴 Eat blanched, steamed, sautéed or grilled
- 🍽️ Tastes great with avocado, black beans, jalapeno pepper, potato or zucchini
- 🧂 Season with cilantro, dill, chili pepper, paprika or tarragon

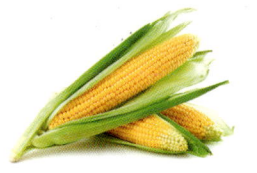

Tip: To remove the kernels from the cob, place the corn cob in a bowl or pan. Run a knife down each side of the corn kernels. The bowl or pan will catch the kernels.

CUCUMBER

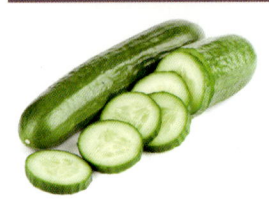

- Choose firm green cucumbers with no soft spots or yellow color.
- Refrigerate sealed in plastic for up to 3 days.
- Wash skin thoroughly with a vegetable brush. Can be peeled before eating.
- Eat raw
- Tastes great with salmon, sour cream, soy sauce, tomato or yogurt
- Season with basil, dill, garlic, lemon or mint

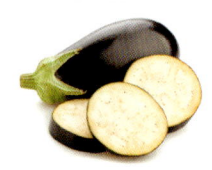

Tip: Cucumbers can replace crackers. Simply slice in circles and top with cheese and dips.

EGGPLANT

- Choose firm eggplant that feels heavy for its size. Skin (purple or white) should be smooth and shiny without cracks or bruises.
- Refrigerate unwashed for 5-7 days.
- Rinse, then cut off ends, peel and slice. It's best to cut right before cooking so it won't turn brown.
- Eat stir-fried or roasted
- Tastes great with bread, mozzarella cheese, tomato or zucchini
- Season with garlic, oregano, parmesan cheese or parsley

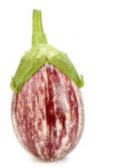

Tip: For tender eggplant, sprinkle 1-inch thick slices with salt, let sit for 30 minutes, rinse with water and pat dry with paper towel.

GREEN BEANS

- Choose bright green, firm beans.
- Refrigerate unwashed in a plastic bag for up to 7 days.
- Rinse and cut or snap off ends.
- Eat raw, blanched, steamed, sautéed or grilled
- Tastes great with almonds, bacon, corn, mushrooms or potato
- Season with mustard, parsley, red pepper flakes or tarragon

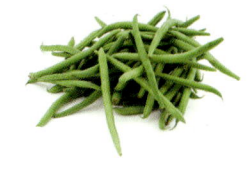

Tip: For a quick side dish, sprinkle steamed green beans with parmesan cheese.

JICAMA

- Choose a jicama that is firm and heavy for its size with no shriveled skin.
- Refrigerate in a plastic bag for up to 2 weeks.
- Scrub under water. Remove skin with knife or peeler.
- Eat raw, blanched, steamed or sautéed
- Tastes great with avocado, orange, cucumber or lettuce
- Season with cilantro, chili powder or hot sauce

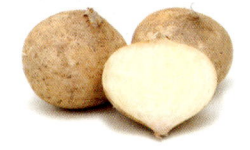

Tip: Peel and slice jicama into "French fry"- sized sticks. Sprinkle with lime juice and a dash of chili powder. Enjoy!

KALE

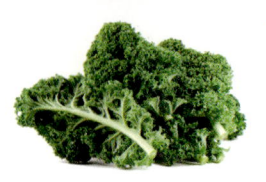

- Choose firm, crisp and deeply colored leaves.
- Refrigerate in an open plastic bag for up to 5 days.
- Rinse, tear off leaves from thick stems. Throw out stems.
- Eat raw, sautéed or baked into crispy chips
- Tastes great with lentils, onion, sausage or tomato
- Season with garlic, lemon or red pepper flakes

Tip: Kale leaves can be sandy. Get rid of sand easily by filling the sink with water, add kale and swish it around. Kale will float and sand will sink.

LETTUCE

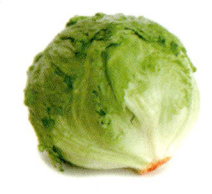

- Choose crisp, closely bunched, bright leaves or heads.
- Refrigerate washed and dried leaves in a plastic bag for up to 1 week.
- Rinse and pat dry with a paper towel or spin dry. Cut or tear off leaves.
- Eat raw
- Tastes great with all vegetables and fruits
- Season with salad dressing, either homemade or store-bought

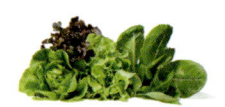

Varieties: Butter, Iceberg, Red and Green Leaf and Romaine

MUSHROOMS

- Choose firm, unblemished caps without mold or wet spots.
- Refrigerate in an open plastic bag or in original store package for up to 1 week.
- Wipe dirt off with a damp cloth. Cut off the end of the stem.
- Eat raw, steamed, sautéed, roasted or grilled
- Tastes great with beef, chicken, egg, green beans, peas, quinoa or rice
- Season with garlic, oregano or parsley

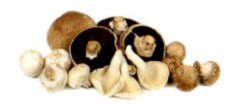

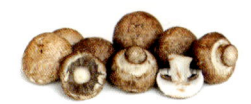

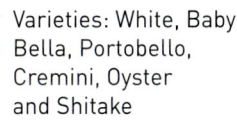

Varieties: White, Baby Bella, Portobello, Cremini, Oyster and Shitake

OKRA

- Choose small to medium sized pods (2-3 inches long) that are deep green, firm, and free of blemishes.
- Refrigerate for up to 3 days.
- Gently scrub under water with a vegetable brush, then slice off ends.
- Eat raw, blanched, steamed, sautéed or roasted
- Tastes great with onions, bell pepper, rice or tomato
- Season with curry powder, garlic or oregano

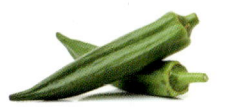

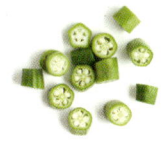

ONION

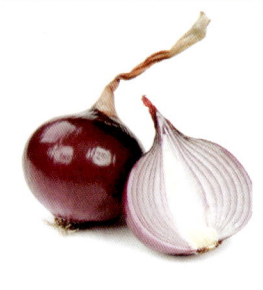

Varieties: Yellow, Red, White, Vidalia and Scallions/Green Onions

- 🛒 Choose firm dry onions with shiny, thin skin with no sprouts at the end or black patches.
- Store in a dry, dark, cool place for up to one month (not in a plastic bag).
- Use a sharp knife to remove skin, then slice, dice or quarter.
- Eat raw, steamed, sautéed, roasted or grilled
- Tastes great with beets, beef, bell pepper, chicken, cucumber, mushrooms or peas
- Season with basil, dill, parsley or sage

PEAS

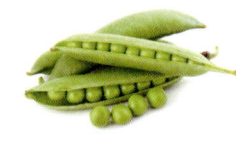

- 🛒 Choose peas that are firm, plump, bright green pods.
- Refrigerate in an open plastic bag for up to 5 days.
- Wash and remove peas from pods. Throw out the pods.
- Eat steamed or sautéed
- Tastes great with carrot, mushrooms, onion, rice or pasta
- Season with dill, lemon, mint, tarragon or thyme

PARSNIP

- Choose small to medium-sized parsnips that are a creamy-white color. They should be firm without any soft spots.
- Refrigerate in an open plastic bag for 3 weeks or more.
- Scrub with vegetable brush, cut off ends and peel with vegetable peeler.
- Eat steamed, stir-fried or roasted
- Tastes great with apple, carrot or potato
- Season with brown sugar, garlic or ginger

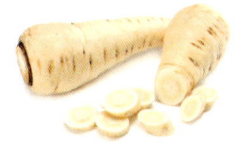

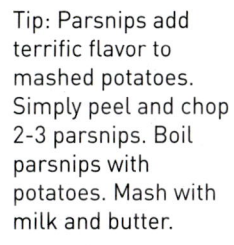

Tip: Parsnips add terrific flavor to mashed potatoes. Simply peel and chop 2-3 parsnips. Boil parsnips with potatoes. Mash with milk and butter.

POTATO

- Choose firm potatoes without green spots or sprouts.
- Store unwashed in a dry, dark, cool place for 3-5 weeks.
- Scrub with a vegetable brush. Cook whole with skin or sliced with or without skin.
- Eat stir-fried, roasted, boiled or baked
- Tastes great with cheese, egg, onion, spinach or peas
- Season with curry powder, parsley, rosemary or thyme

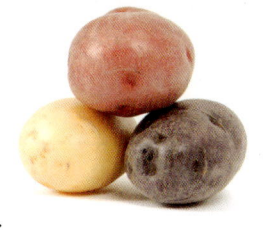

Varieties: Russet, Idaho, Red, Blue, New, White, Yukon Gold and Fingerling

RADISH

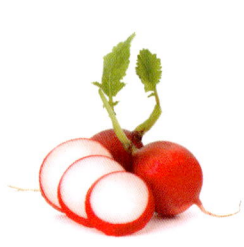

🛒 Choose radishes that are firm and brightly colored. If the radishes have the leaves on, avoid greens that are limp or wilted.

❄️ Remove greens. Refrigerate radishes in a plastic bag for up to 1 week.

🔪 Wash well and trim the ends.

🍴 Eat raw or roasted

🍽️ Tastes great with carrot, celery, cucumber, lettuce or tomato

🧂 Season with chives, cilantro, dill or lemon

Tip: To soften the peppery flavor of radishes, roast them to bring out their sweetness with a little olive oil and salt.

SPINACH

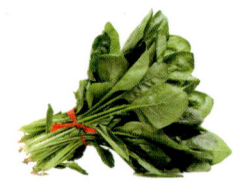

🛒 Choose crisp, dark green, even-colored leaves.

❄️ Refrigerate washed and loosely wrapped in paper towel for up to 5 days.

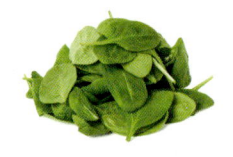

🔪 Soak in cold water and swish leaves to remove sand and dirt. Pat dry with paper towels.

🍴 Eat raw, steamed or stir-fried

🍽️ Tastes great with fish, mushrooms, potato, sweet potato or white beans

🧂 Season with garlic, ginger, red pepper flakes or salad dressing

Tip: Spinach adds a nutrition boost to a smoothie without changing the flavor.

SWEET POTATO & YAMS

- Sweet potatoes should be firm, smooth shaped and have clean skin.
- Store unwashed in a dry, dark, cool place for 3-5 weeks.
- Scrub well under cold water and remove skin with vegetable peeler. If roasting or baking whole, keep the skin on.
- Eat stir-fried, baked, roasted or grilled
- Tastes great with carrot, ham, lime, nuts or pineapple
- Season with chili pepper, cinnamon, curry powder or maple syrup

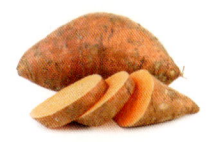

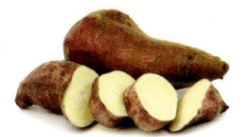

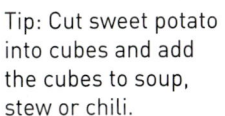

Tip: Cut sweet potato into cubes and add the cubes to soup, stew or chili.

SUGAR SNAP PEAS

- Choose snap peas with firm, shiny, bright green pods.
- Refrigerate in an open plastic bag for up to 2 days.
- Wash and trim both ends.
- Eat raw, blanched, steamed, stir-fried, or grilled
- Tastes great with carrot, mushrooms, onion, pasta or rice
- Season with dill, lemon, mint, soy sauce or tarragon

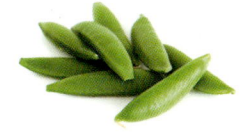

Tip: Sugar snap peas dipped in ranch dressing are a crunchy and healthy snack.

TOMATILLO

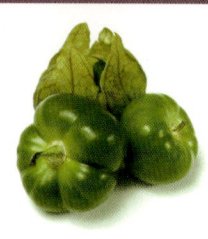

- Choose pale green, firm tomatillos with a crisp, papery husk loosely attached.
- Refrigerate in an open container for up to 3 weeks.
- Remove husk and rinse well.
- Eat raw, roasted or grilled
- Tastes great with avocado, bell pepper, black beans or onion
- Season with cilantro, lime or sweet salad dressing

TOMATO

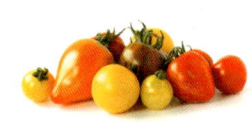

- Choose tomatoes with a fresh smell, even-colored skin and firm texture.
- Store at room temperature for up to 1 week.
- Wash and remove core with a knife.
- Eat raw, roasted or grilled
- Tastes great with avocado, cheese, chickpeas, egg, onion or pasta
- Season with basil, garlic, oregano or salad dressing

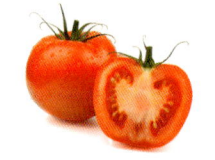

Varieties: Beefsteak, Heirloom, Cherry, Grape, Plum/Roma

WINTER SQUASH

- Choose winter squash that are heavy for their size with a deep colored skin.
- Store unwashed in a cool, dark place for up to 1 month.
- Wash and cut in half, scoop out seeds. Discard seeds. Peel with a vegetable peeler or leave skin on for baking large pieces.
- Eat steamed, sautéed, roasted or grilled
- Tastes great with apples, broccoli, corn, rice, sausage or spinach
- Season with cinnamon, cloves, curry powder, maple syrup or sage

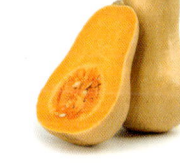

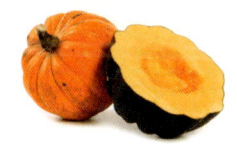

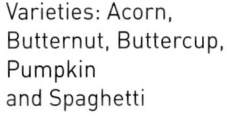

Varieties: Acorn, Butternut, Buttercup, Pumpkin and Spaghetti

ZUCCHINI

- Choose smaller sized squash that are dark green, firm and smooth skinned.
- Refrigerate in an open plastic bag for up to 5 days.
- Rinse and trim ends.
- Eat raw, blanched, steamed, sautéed, roasted or grilled
- Tastes great with bell peppers, corn, eggplant or tomato
- Season with basil, garlic, parmesan cheese or oregano

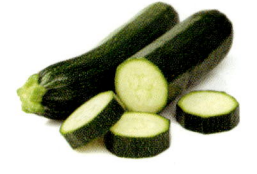

Tip: Add shredded zucchini to a brownie or chocolate cake recipe. It will add a boost of nutrition, but won't change the flavor.

How to steam vegetables

Steaming vegetables on the stovetop or in the microwave is fast and easy. Season steamed vegetables with fresh chopped herbs, a pinch of salt and pepper or a dash of no-salt herb blend. Toss the seasoned vegetables with a little olive oil or butter and serve!

Stovetop steaming what you need:

Ingredients

- Vegetables
- Water

Tools

- Cutting board and knife
- Pot with lid
- Steamer basket

Instructions

1. Prepare vegetables by cutting them into same-size pieces.
2. Wash vegetables in cold water.
3. Add 1 inch of water to a pot. Set the vegetables in the steamer basket
4. Bring the water to a boil then cover and reduce heat to a medium. Steam the vegetables for a few minutes. Vegetables are done when their color is bright, and they have a slight crunch.
5. Remove from heat, season and serve.

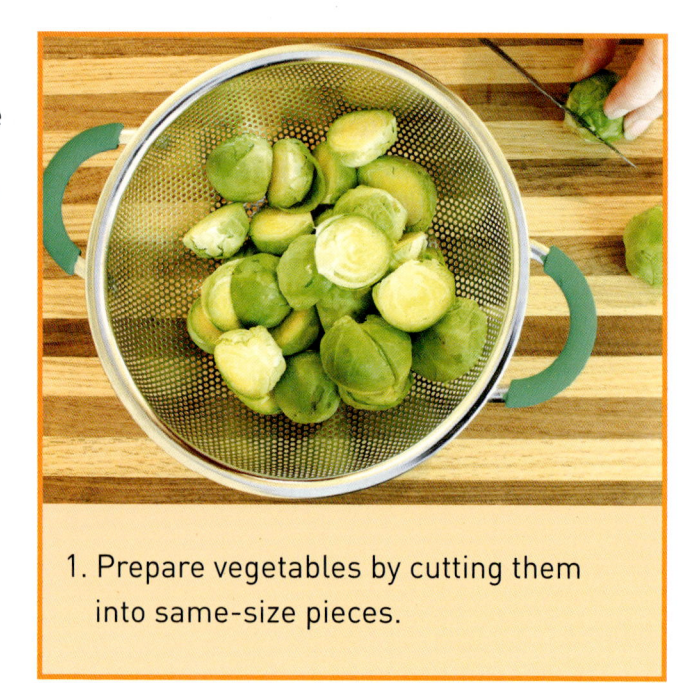

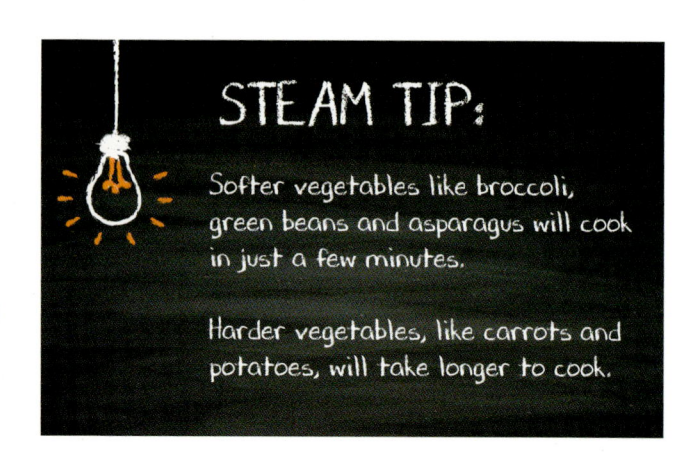

1. Prepare vegetables by cutting them into same-size pieces.

STEAM TIP:

Softer vegetables like broccoli, green beans and asparagus will cook in just a few minutes.

Harder vegetables, like carrots and potatoes, will take longer to cook.

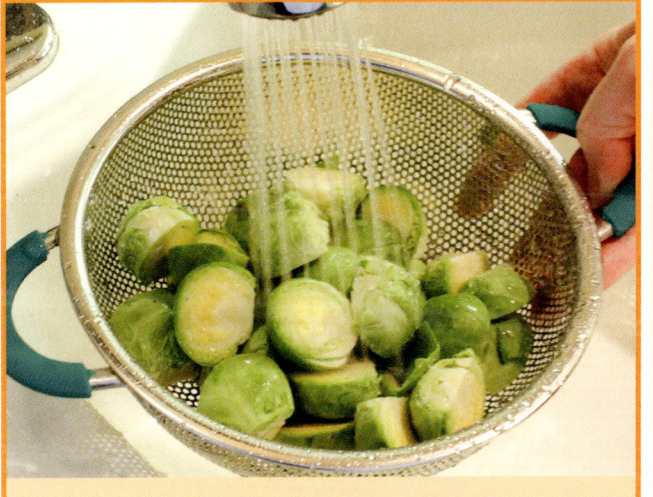

2. Wash vegetables in cold water.

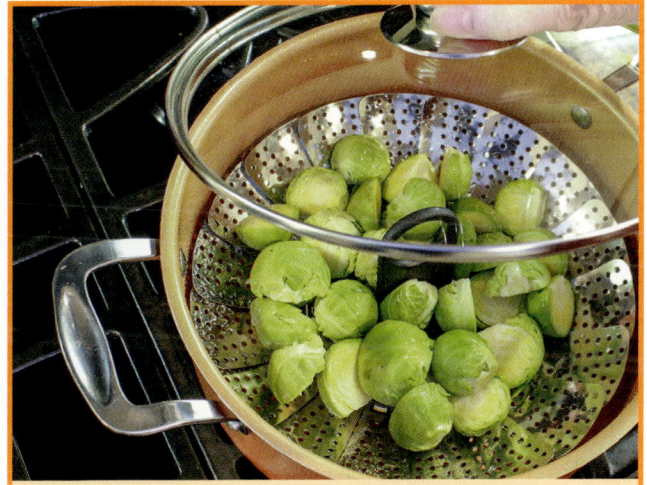

3. Add 1-inch of water to pot. Set the vegetables in the steamer basket.

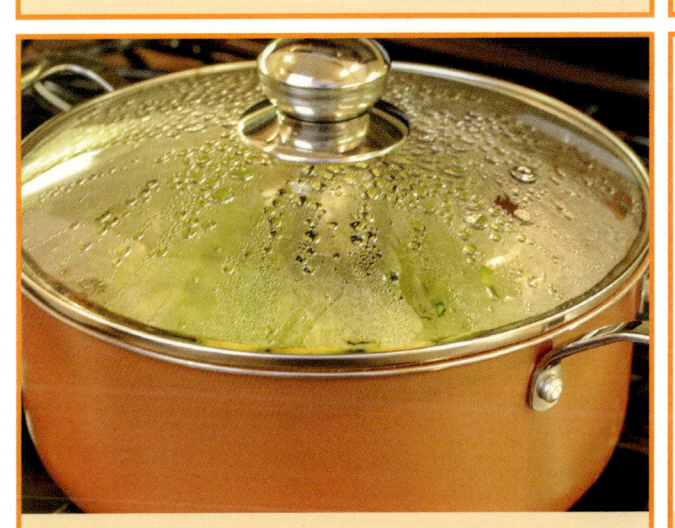

4. Bring to a boil. Cover and reduce heat to medium.

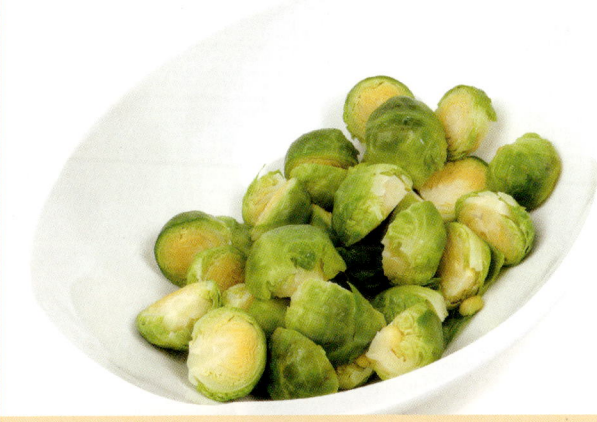

5. Remove from heat, season and serve.

Microwave steaming what you need:

Ingredients

- Vegetables
- Water

Tools

- Cutting board and knife
- Microwave-safe dish
- Microwave-safe plastic wrap

Instructions

1. Prepare vegetables and cut them into same-sized pieces.
2. Wash vegetables in cold water.
3. Place vegetables in a microwave-safe bowl with a little water added. Cover the bowl with plastic wrap, poke 2-3 holes in the plastic wrap with a knife. This helps steam escape.
4. Microwave vegetables on high, most will cook in about 3-4 minutes (depending on the power of the microwave and how many vegetables you cook). Vegetables are done when their color is bright, and they have a slight crunch.
5. Remove the bowl from the microwave with a potholder. Remove the plastic wrap, being careful of hot steam escaping. Season vegetables and serve.

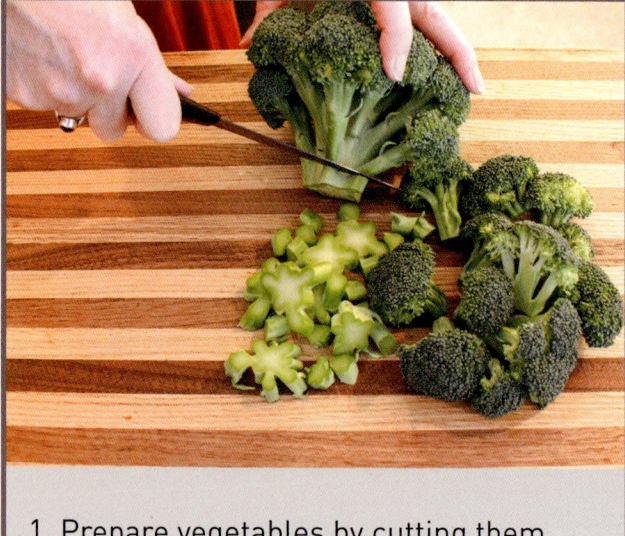

1. Prepare vegetables by cutting them into same-size pieces.

2. Wash vegetables in cold water.

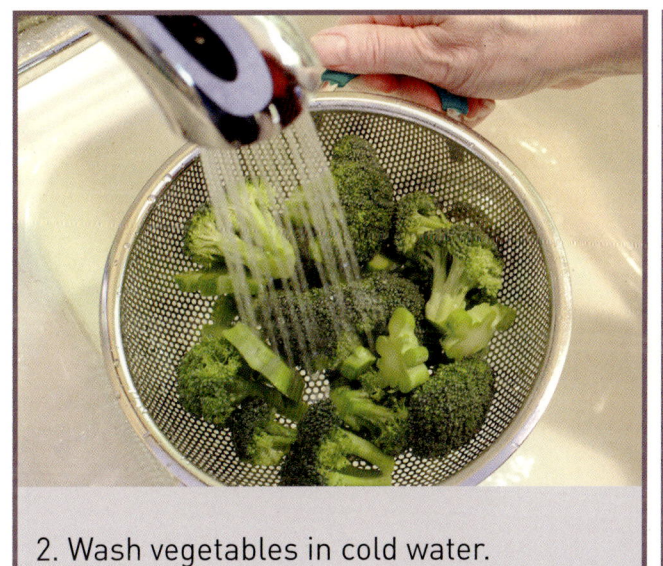

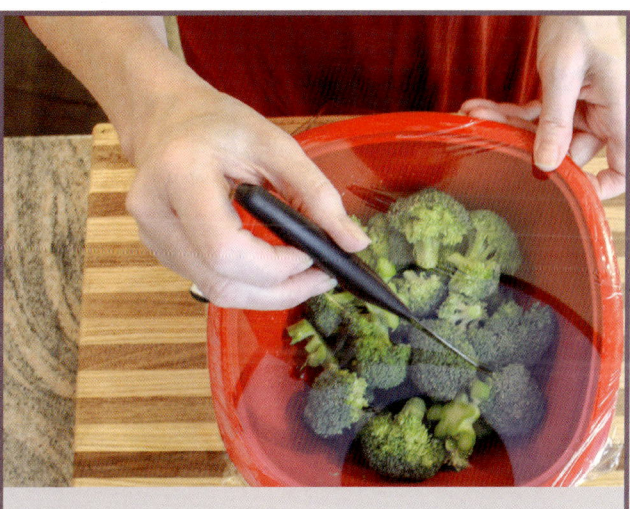

3. Cover the bowl with plastic wrap, poke 2-3 holes in the plastic wrap with a knife.

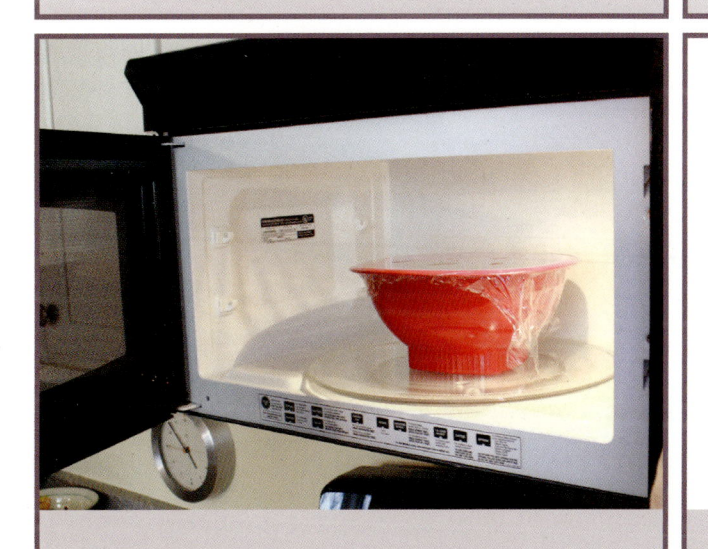

4. Microwave vegetables on HIGH. Most vegetables will cook in 3-4 minutes.

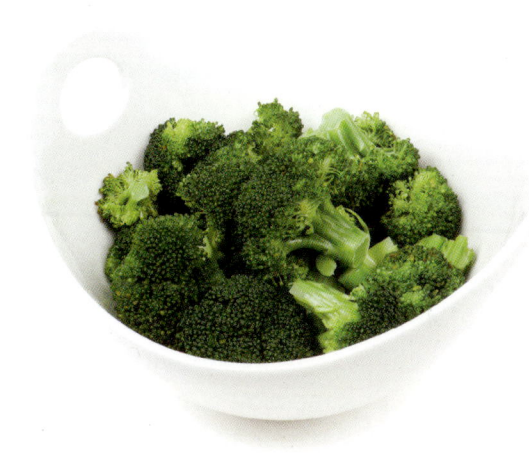

5. Remove the bowl from the microwave. Season and serve.

How to roast vegetables:

Roasted vegetables are packed with flavor and crisp on the outside and moist and tender on the inside. Roasting vegetables is as easy as putting them in the oven.

What you need:

Ingredients

- 3 - 4 cups of any vegetable
- 1-2 Tbsp vegetable oil
- 1 tsp salt
- ¼ tsp black pepper

Tools

- Cutting board and knife
- Mixing bowl
- Measuring spoons
- Spatula
- Baking sheet
- Aluminum foil or parchment paper (optional, but makes clean up easy!)

1. Preheat the oven to 425°F. Wash vegetables.

Instructions

1. Preheat the oven to 425°F with a rack in the middle position. Wash and dry vegetables.
2. Cut vegetables into the same-size chunks or pieces.
3. In a mixing bowl, toss the vegetables with oil, salt and pepper.
4. Spread the vegetables onto a baking sheet (lined with foil or parchment paper) in a single layer. If the vegetables are too crowded, they will steam instead of roast.
5. Place the pan in the oven and roast the vegetables until fork tender and showing brown crispy tips and edges. Serve right away.

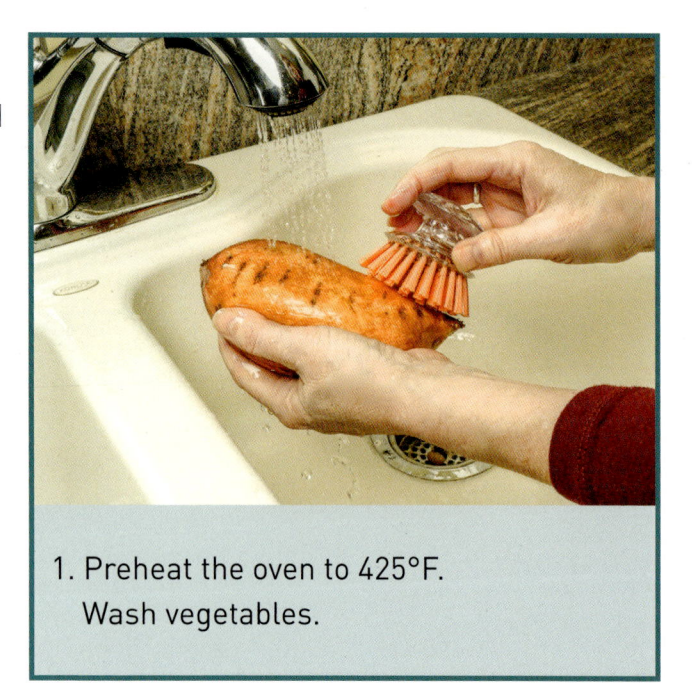

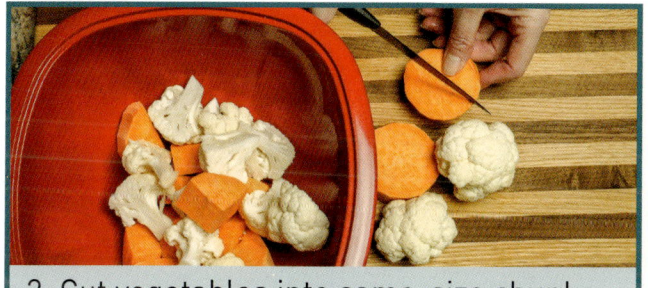

2. Cut vegetables into same-size chunks or pieces.

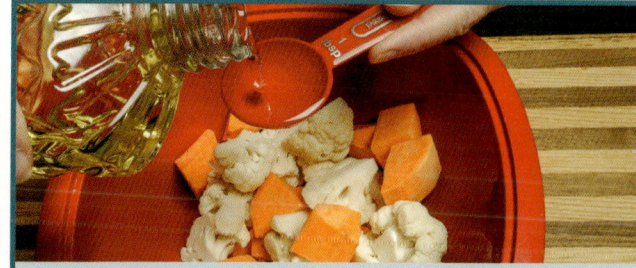

3. In a mixing bowl, toss the vegetables with oil, salt and pepper.

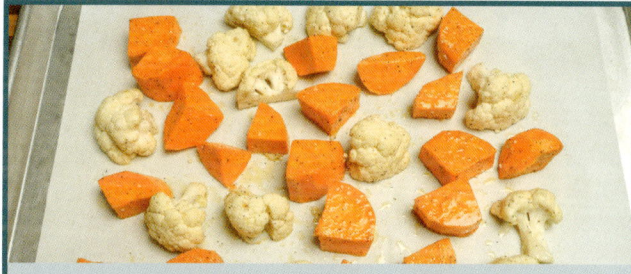

4. Spread the vegetables onto a baking sheet in a single layer.

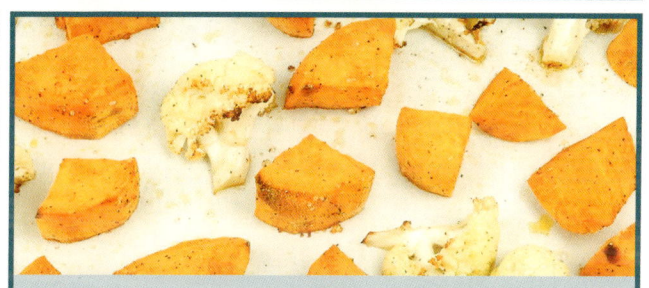

5. Roast the vegetables until fork tender with brown crispy edges. Serve right away.

Vegetable	Cooking Time
Acorn squash, butternut squash, beets, carrots, cauliflower, onions, parsnips, potatoes, yams	40-45 minutes
Broccoli, brussels sprouts, eggplant, mushrooms	25-30 minutes
Asparagus, bell peppers, green beans, summer squash, tomatoes, zucchini	15-20 minutes

Tip for roasting a mix of vegetables

Add different vegetables to the baking sheet at different times. Start with the longest-cooking vegetables first, and then add quicker-cooking vegetables later. If the baking sheet gets full, split the vegetables between two pans so you don't overcrowd them.

How much do I need for a recipe?

Many recipes call for vegetables in cups or ounces, but that's not how they are sold at the market. Use this helpful table to buy the amount of fresh vegetables needed for a recipe.

Example: If a recipe calls for 1 cup of chopped carrots, you will need about 3 medium carrots.

Vegetable	Recipe calls for	Fresh Equivalent
Asparagus	2 cups, trimmed and chopped	19-20 medium spears
Bell pepper	1/2 cup, chopped	1 medium
Broccoli	3 1/2 cups florets	1 medium head
Cabbage	8 cups, shredded	1 medium head
Carrots	1 cup, shredded, chopped or sliced	3 medium
Cauliflower	3 cups	1 medium head
Celery	1/2 cup, sliced	1 medium stalk
Collard greens	1 1/2 cups, cooked	6-7 cups, uncooked
Corn on the cob	1 cup kernels	1-2 ears
Cucumber	1 cup, peeled, seeded and diced	1 medium
Eggplant	4 1/2 cups, cubed	1 medium
Green onions	2 Tbsp, chopped	1 medium stalk
Herbs (dill, basil, ginger, oregano)	1 tsp, dried	1 Tablespoon, fresh
Lemon	2 Tbsp juice	1 medium
Lettuce (Iceberg)	4 cups, shredded; 6-8 cups, torn	1 medium head
Lime	2 Tbsp juice	1 medium
Mushrooms	1 6-8 oz. can; 1 pound (16 oz.), sliced or chopped	20-24 mushrooms
Onion powder	1 Tbsp	1 medium onion, chopped
Onions	1 cup, chopped	1 small onion
Parsnips	2 cups, diced	4 medium
Radishes	1/2 cup, thinly sliced	5-6 radishes
Spinach	1 1/2 cups, cooked	4 cups torn leaves
Sweet potatoes	2/3 cup, cubed; 3/4 cup, sliced; 1/2 cup, cooked and mashed	1 medium
Swiss chard	2 1/2 cups, cooked	9-10 cups, raw
Tomatoes (Plum/Roma)	1 cup, chopped	3 medium
Tomatoes (Round)	1 cup, chopped	1 large
Zucchini	2/3 cup grated, 1 cup sliced	1 medium

Recipe List		
Breakfasts	Avocado Egg Toast Broccoli and Ham Breakfast Bake Green Smoothie Pumpkin Pancakes Veggie Oatmeal Bowl	
Salsas, sauces and dips	Avocado Hummus Corn Relish Cucumber Yogurt Sauce Fresh Tomato Salsa	
Soups	Broccoli Cheese Soup Minestrone Soup Roasted Squash and Garlic Soup Southwestern Tortilla Soup Spinach Ginger Soup	
Salads	Black Bean, Corn and Tomato Salad Ramen Noodle Slaw MyPlate-Style Tossed Salad Carrot Pineapple Salad	
Sides	Creamed Spinach Baked Sweet Potatoes Fried Rice-Style Quinoa Candied Brussel Sprouts and Carrots Green Beans, Corn and Bacon Stir and Serve Mushrooms Kale Chips	
Main dishes	Pan Roasted Chicken and Vegetables Sweet Potato Burritos with Avocado Crema Zucchini Lasagna Creamy Pasta Primavera	

How to tackle a recipe

Recipes are written in two parts. There is a list of ingredients and then a set of directions. For best results, follow these tips:

1. Read the recipe all the way through before you start.

2. Check your supplies to make sure you have all the ingredients.

3. See that you have the right equipment for the recipe.

4. When you are ready to get started, get out all the ingredients and the equipment.

5. Follow the recipe instructions. Measure ingredients and follow cooking times.

Tbsp = Tablespoon
tsp = teaspoon
oz. = ounces

BREAKFAST

Avocado Egg Toast
Serves 1

Ingredients:

1 slice of whole grain bread, toasted
½ avocado, mashed
1 egg
Cooking spray

Directions:

1. Mash avocado in a small bowl.
2. Heat a small nonstick skillet over low heat, spray with cooking spray and gently crack the egg into it. Cook the egg until the whites are no longer clear and yolk is still soft.
3. Spread mashed avocado on the toast, top with egg. Serve.

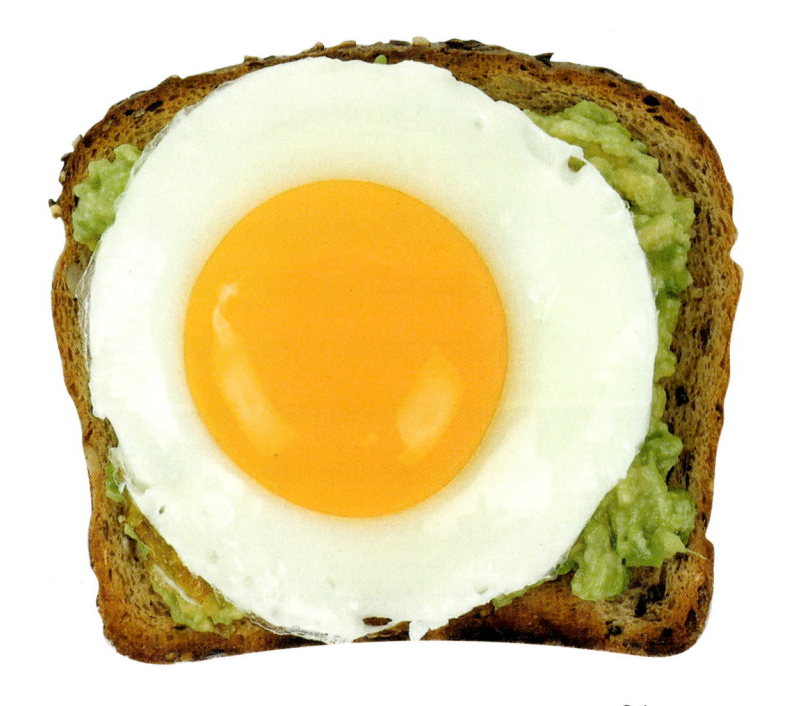

Nutrition Facts	
Serving size	1
Amount Per Serving	
Calories	**260**
	% Daily Value*
Total Fat 18g	23%
Saturated Fat 3.5g	18%
Trans Fat 0.5g	
Cholesterol 185mg	62%
Sodium 160mg	7%
Total Carbohydrate 18g	7%
Dietary Fiber 7g	25%
Total Sugars 2g	
Includes 0g Added Sugars	0%
Protein 10g	
Vitamin D 0mcg	0%
Calcium 60mg	4%
Iron 1.9mg	10%
Potassium 500mg	10%

* The % Daily Value (DV) tells you how much a nutrient in a serving of food contributes to a daily diet. 2,000 calories a day is used for general nutrition advice.

Broccoli and Ham Breakfast Bake
Serves 6

Ingredients:

6 large eggs
½ cup 2% lowfat milk
¾ cup ham, diced
1 cup broccoli, chopped
½ cup frozen sweet corn
½ cup cheddar cheese, shredded
1 Tbsp butter

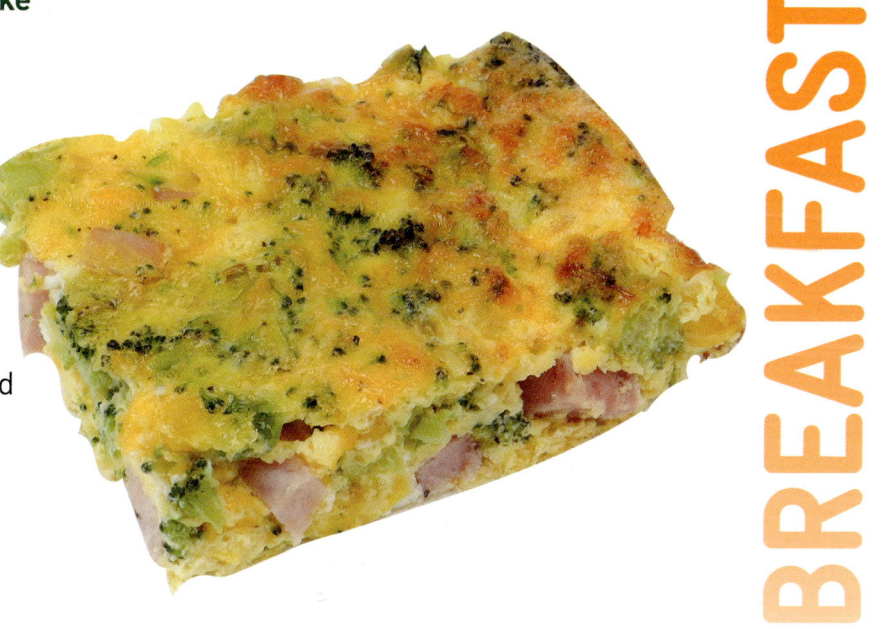

Directions:

1. Preheat oven to 350°F. Place a 9x9-inch baking dish in the oven to warm.
2. While the oven heats up, beat the eggs in a bowl and stir in the rest of the ingredients.
3. Pull the baking dish out of the oven. Spread the butter around the bottom and up the sides of the pan.
4. Pour egg mixture into the dish.
5. Bake for approximately 20 minutes until center is dry.

Tip: Freeze leftover pieces. Defrost and warm in the microwave for an easy morning breakfast.

Nutrition Facts

6 servings per recipe
Serving size 1/6

Amount Per Serving
Calories 160

	% Daily Value*
Total Fat 11g	14%
Saturated Fat 5g	25%
Trans Fat 1g	
Cholesterol 210mg	70%
Sodium 330mg	14%
Total Carbohydrate 6g	2%
Dietary Fiber <1g	2%
Total Sugars 2g	
Includes 0g Added Sugars	0%
Protein 12g	
Vitamin D 0.2mcg	2%
Calcium 130mg	10%
Iron 1.1mg	6%
Potassium 170mg	4%

* The % Daily Value (DV) tells you how much a nutrient in a serving of food contributes to a daily diet. 2,000 calories a day is used for general nutrition advice.

BREAKFAST

BREAKFAST

Green Smoothie
Serves 2 (makes 2 - 8 oz. servings)

Ingredients:

1 ripe medium banana, peeled
1 apple, peeled and core removed
1 cup spinach leaves, tough stems removed
¼ cup cold orange juice
¼ cup cold 2% lowfat milk
6 ice cubes

Directions:

1. Chop apple and spinach leaves.
2. Place banana, apple, spinach, orange juice, milk and ice cubes in a blender. Pulse a few times, then puree until smooth, scraping down the sides as necessary.

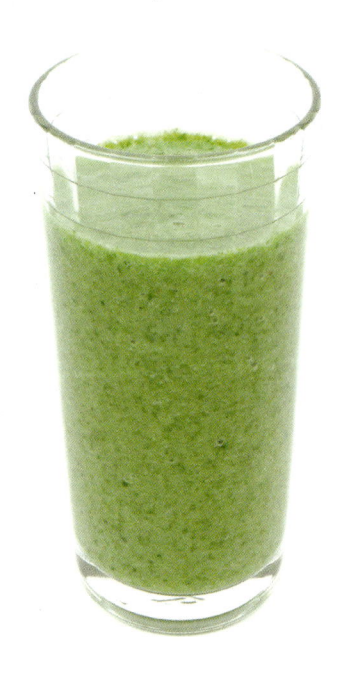

Nutrition Facts
2 servings per recipe

Serving size	**8 ounce**

Amount Per Serving

Calories 150

	% Daily Value*
Total Fat 1.5g	**2%**
Saturated Fat 0g	**0%**
Trans Fat 0g	
Cholesterol <5mg	**1%**
Sodium 75mg	**3%**
Total Carbohydrate 33g	**12%**
Dietary Fiber 5g	**18%**
Total Sugars 20g	
Includes 3g Added Sugars	**6%**
Protein 5g	
Vitamin D 0.3mcg	2%
Calcium 150mg	10%
Iron 1.7mg	10%
Potassium 620mg	15%

* The % Daily Value (DV) tells you how much a nutrient in a serving of food contributes to a daily diet. 2,000 calories a day is used for general nutrition advice.

Pumpkin Pancakes
Serves 4 (makes 12 - 3" pancakes)

Ingredients:

2 cups pancake mix
1 cup 2% lowfat milk
1 egg
½ cup canned pumpkin puree
2 Tbsp sugar
½ tsp ground cinnamon

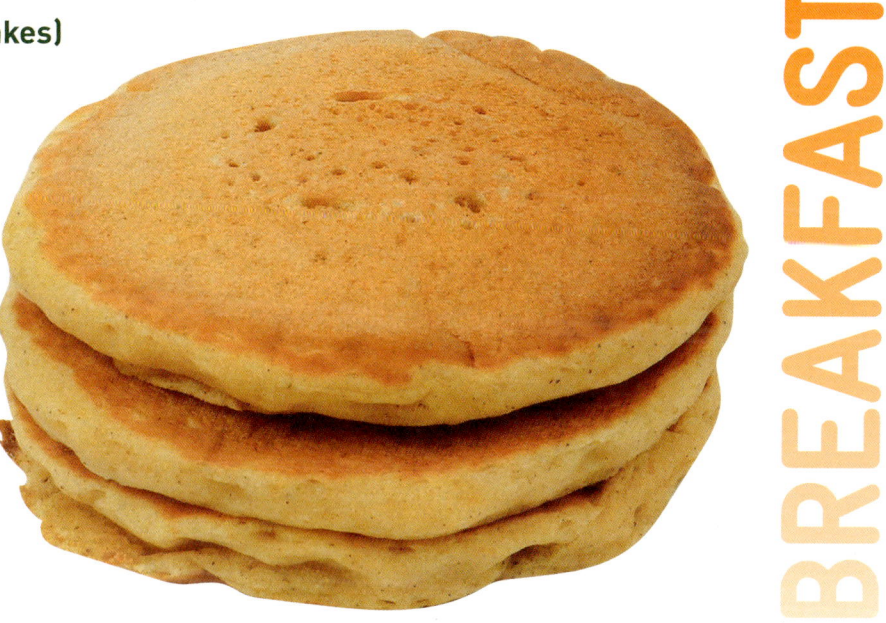

BREAKFAST

Directions:

1. In a medium/large bowl, combine all the ingredients until just blended (batter can be a little lumpy).
2. Spray skillet pan with nonstick spray and heat over medium heat. Spoon ¼ cup of batter into pan to form each pancake. Cook until edges are drying and bubbles start to pop.
3. Using a flat spatula, turn each pancake over and cook 2-3 minutes longer.
4. Serve with maple syrup and banana slices.

Nutrition Facts

4 servings per recipe

Serving size	3 pancakes

Amount Per Serving

Calories 290

	% Daily Value*
Total Fat 3.5g	4%
Saturated Fat 1g	5%
Trans Fat 0g	
Cholesterol 50mg	17%
Sodium 510mg	22%
Total Carbohydrate 54g	20%
Dietary Fiber 11g	39%
Total Sugars 13g	
Includes 6g Added Sugars	12%
Protein 12g	
Vitamin D 0.6mcg	4%
Calcium 180mg	15%
Iron 4mg	20%
Potassium 130mg	2%

* The % Daily Value (DV) tells you how much a nutrient in a serving of food contributes to a daily diet. 2,000 calories a day is used for general nutrition advice.

BREAKFAST

Veggie Oatmeal Bowl
Serves 1

Ingredients:

½ cup oatmeal (quick or old fashioned), uncooked
1 cup 2% lowfat milk
½ cup baby spinach leaves, long stems removed
¼ cup tomatoes, chopped
1 Tbsp part-skim mozzarella cheese, shredded

Directions:

1. Make oatmeal according to the package directions. Use milk instead of water.
2. Chop the spinach leaves. Stir the spinach into the hot oatmeal.
3. Spoon the oatmeal into a bowl. Top with the shredded cheese and chopped tomato.
4. Season to taste with salt, pepper or hot sauce.

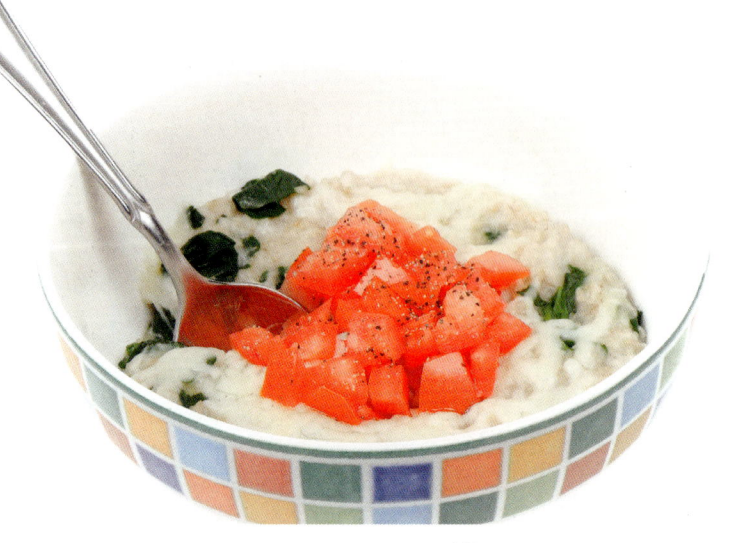

Nutrition Facts

1 serving per recipe
Serving size 1

Amount Per Serving
Calories 340

	% Daily Value*
Total Fat 9g	12%
Saturated Fat 4g	20%
Trans Fat 0g	
Cholesterol 25mg	8%
Sodium 250mg	11%
Total Carbohydrate 46g	17%
Dietary Fiber 7g	25%
Total Sugars 15g	
Includes 0g Added Sugars	0%
Protein 20g	
Vitamin D 2.5mcg	10%
Calcium 530mg	40%
Iron 3.5mg	20%
Potassium 980mg	20%

* The % Daily Value (DV) tells you how much a nutrient in a serving of food contributes to a daily diet. 2,000 calories a day is used for general nutrition advice.

Broccoli Cheese Soup
Serves 6 (1 cup servings)

Ingredients:

6 cups broccoli, chopped
4 Tbsp butter
1 cup onion, minced
½ cup celery, minced
½ cup carrots, minced
2 Tbsp flour
2 cups, (16 oz.) low-sodium chicken broth
2 cups 2% lowfat milk
4 cups (1 lb.) mild cheddar cheese, shredded

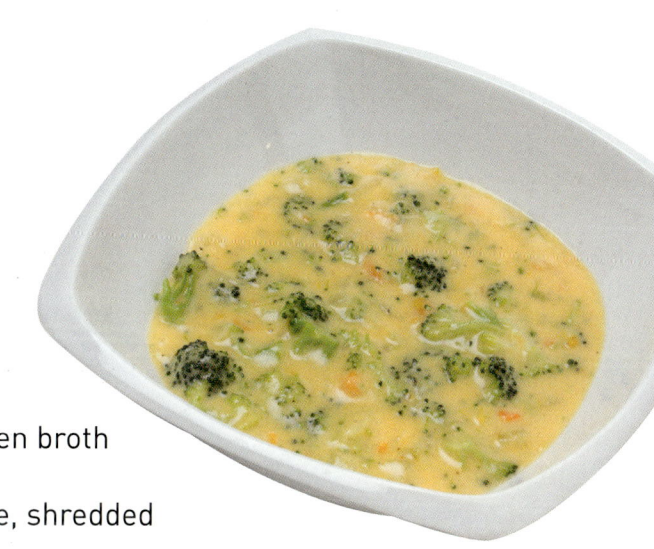

Directions:

1. Steam broccoli in a covered, microwave-safe dish for 3 minutes. Drain off any water from cooking.
2. Melt butter in a large pot over medium heat. Add onions, carrots, and celery. Cover and cook for 8 minutes until vegetables are soft.
3. Stir in flour to coat the vegetables, keep stirring and cook for 1 minute.
4. Slowly add the chicken broth and milk, stirring constantly. Cook for 5 minutes, stirring occasionally.
5. Add cheese, let stand for 1 minute, then stir to combine the cheese with the soup broth. Warm soup for 3 minutes, but do not let it boil.
6. Add broccoli and warm for one more minute. Season with salt and pepper.

Tip: If the soup is too thick, thin it by adding milk.

Nutrition Facts

6 servings per recipe
Serving size: 1 cup

Amount Per Serving
Calories 80

	% Daily Value*
Total Fat 6g	8%
Saturated Fat 3.5g	18%
Trans Fat 0g	
Cholesterol 20mg	7%
Sodium 110mg	5%
Total Carbohydrate 3g	1%
Dietary Fiber <1g	2%
Total Sugars 1g	
Includes 0g Added Sugars	0%
Protein 5g	
Vitamin D 0.2mcg	0%
Calcium 120mg	10%
Iron 0.2mg	2%
Potassium 90mg	2%

* The % Daily Value (DV) tells you how much a nutrient in a serving of food contributes to a daily diet. 2,000 calories a day is used for general nutrition advice.

SOUPS

Minestrone Soup
Serves 6 (1 cup servings)

Ingredients:

2 Tbsp vegetable oil
3 garlic cloves, minced
½ cup carrot, diced
½ cup onion, diced
½ cup celery, diced
¼ head cabbage
1 can (14 oz.) garbanzo beans, drained and rinsed
1 can (14 oz.) diced tomatoes
4 cups (32 oz.) low-sodium chicken broth
1 cup elbow pasta
1 tsp Italian seasoning

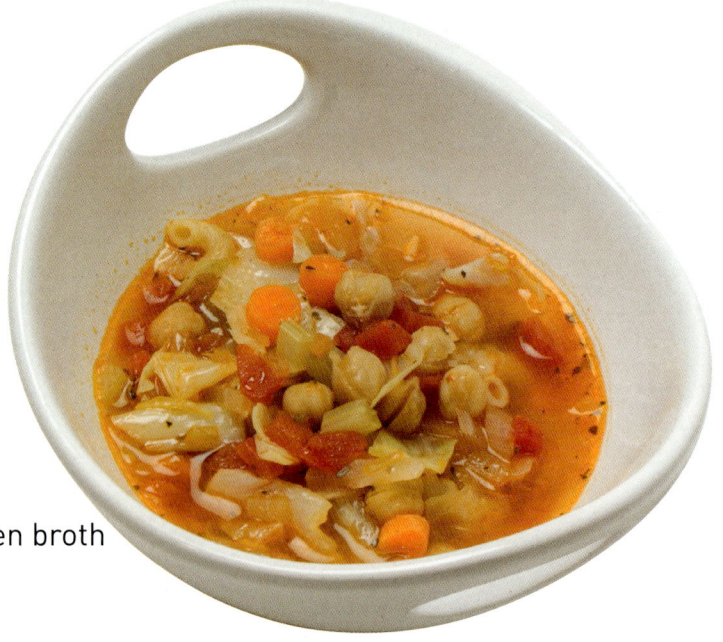

Directions:

1. Chop cabbage into 1-inch size pieces.
2. Heat oil in large soup pot on medium heat, add garlic, carrot, onion, celery and cabbage and cook for 8 minutes until the vegetables are soft.
3. Add garbanzo beans, diced tomatoes, pasta, seasoning and chicken broth. Bring to a boil. Turn heat down to low and simmer 15 minutes.

Nutrition Facts

6 servings per recipe

Serving size	**1 cup**

Amount Per Serving

Calories 45

	% Daily Value*
Total Fat 1.5g	2%
Saturated Fat 0.5g	3%
Trans Fat 0g	
Cholesterol 0mg	0%
Sodium 55mg	2%
Total Carbohydrate 6g	2%
Dietary Fiber 1g	4%
Total Sugars 1g	
Includes 0g Added Sugars	0%
Protein 2g	
Vitamin D 0mcg	0%
Calcium 10mg	2%
Iron 0.4mg	2%
Potassium 80mg	2%

* The % Daily Value (DV) tells you how much a nutrient in a serving of food contributes to a daily diet. 2,000 calories a day is used for general nutrition advice.

Roasted Squash and Garlic Soup
Serves 6 (1 cup servings)

Ingredients:

1 large or 2 small butternut squash
10 garlic cloves, peeled
2 Tbsp vegetable oil
¼ cup water
4 cups (32 oz.) low-sodium chicken broth
1½ cups 2% lowfat milk
1 Tbsp lemon juice (about ½ lemon)

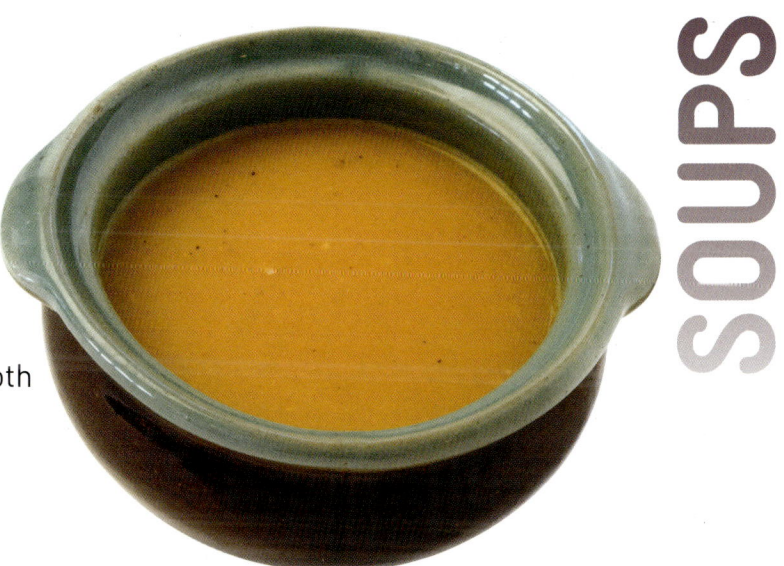

SOUPS

Directions:

1. Preheat oven to 400°F.
2. Cut the squash in half and remove seeds and fibers. Using a vegetable peeler, peel off the squash skin and cut the squash into 1-inch thick slices.
3. Place the squash and garlic cloves in a roasting pan. Sprinkle with salt and pepper. Drizzle with oil and toss with a spoon until well coated. Pour in the water. Put the pan in the oven.
4. Roast the squash and garlic, about 45 minutes. Check the squash while its cooking, if the pan looks dry, add water. The squash is done if a fork slides easily into it. Remove it from the oven and set aside to cool for 5 minutes.
5. Place about half of the roasted squash and garlic with 1 cup of the chicken broth in a blender. Puree until smooth. Transfer the puree to a large soup pan. Process the rest of the squash and garlic the same way. Stir in the remaining soup stock, milk, and lemon juice.
6. To serve, warm soup and ladle into bowls.

Nutrition Facts

6 servings per recipe

Serving size	**1 cup**

Amount Per Serving

Calories 25

	% Daily Value*
Total Fat 1g	1%
Saturated Fat 1g	5%
Trans Fat 0g	
Cholesterol 0mg	0%
Sodium 15mg	1%
Total Carbohydrate 3g	1%
Dietary Fiber 0g	0%
Total Sugars <1g	
Includes 0g Added Sugars	0%
Protein 1g	
Vitamin D 0.1mcg	0%
Calcium 20mg	2%
Iron 0.1mg	0%
Potassium 90mg	2%

* The % Daily Value (DV) tells you how much a nutrient in a serving of food contributes to a daily diet. 2,000 calories a day is used for general nutrition advice.

SOUPS

Southwestern Tortilla Soup
Serves 6 (1 cup servings)

Ingredients:

4 cups (32 oz.) low-sodium chicken broth
1 can (14 oz.) diced tomatoes, southwestern flavored
1 can (4 oz.) chopped green chiles
1 can (14 oz.) black beans, drained and rinsed
½ cup frozen corn
2 cups cooked chicken, diced or shredded
2 Tbsp lime juice (about 2 limes)
2 Tbsp cilantro, chopped
Tortilla chips, crushed into smaller pieces

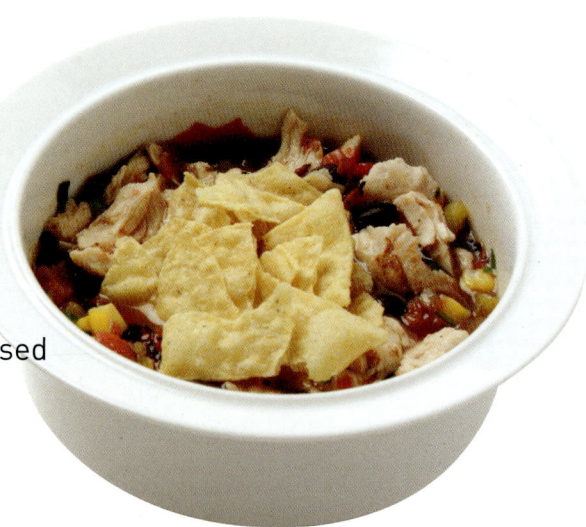

Directions:

1. In a large soup pot, add chicken broth, tomatoes, green chiles, black beans, corn, and chicken. Over medium-high heat, bring to a boil. Reduce heat to low and simmer for 5 minutes.
2. Turn off heat. Stir in lime juice and cilantro.
3. Spoon the soup in to bowls. Serve with tortilla chips.

Nutrition Facts
6 servings per recipe

Serving size	1 cup

Amount Per Serving
Calories 210

	% Daily Value*
Total Fat 3g	4%
Saturated Fat 1g	5%
Trans Fat 0g	
Cholesterol 65mg	22%
Sodium 350mg	15%
Total Carbohydrate 20g	7%
Dietary Fiber 6g	21%
Total Sugars 2g	
Includes 0g Added Sugars	0%
Protein 26g	
Vitamin D 0mcg	0%
Calcium 60mg	4%
Iron 2.6mg	15%
Potassium 720mg	15%

* The % Daily Value (DV) tells you how much a nutrient in a serving of food contributes to a daily diet. 2,000 calories a day is used for general nutrition advice.

Spinach Ginger Soup
Serves 6 (1 cup servings)

Ingredients:

2 Tbsp vegetable oil
1 onion, chopped
2 garlic cloves, minced
1-inch piece of ginger, minced
1 bag (10 oz.) spinach, long stems removed
1 medium potato, peeled and chopped
4 cups (32 oz.) low-sodium chicken broth
1 can (14 oz.) coconut milk
Salt and pepper

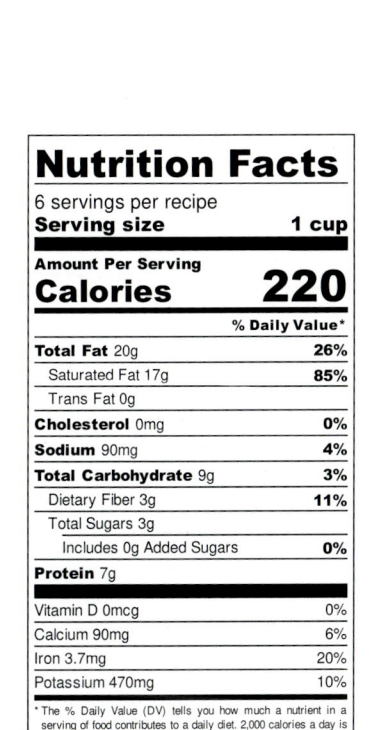

SOUPS

Nutrition Facts

6 servings per recipe
Serving size 1 cup

Amount Per Serving
Calories 220

	% Daily Value*
Total Fat 20g	26%
Saturated Fat 17g	85%
Trans Fat 0g	
Cholesterol 0mg	0%
Sodium 90mg	4%
Total Carbohydrate 9g	3%
Dietary Fiber 3g	11%
Total Sugars 3g	
Includes 0g Added Sugars	0%
Protein 7g	
Vitamin D 0mcg	0%
Calcium 90mg	6%
Iron 3.7mg	20%
Potassium 470mg	10%

* The % Daily Value (DV) tells you how much a nutrient in a serving of food contributes to a daily diet. 2,000 calories a day is used for general nutrition advice.

Directions:

1. Heat the oil in a large saucepan over medium heat. Add the onion, garlic and ginger and cook until softened but not brown, about 3-4 minutes.
2. Add spinach to the pan. Stir until spinach is wilted.
3. Add the broth and potato and bring to a boil. Lower heat, cover and simmer 10-15 minutes. Let cool for 10 minutes.
4. Pour soup into blender and process until smooth. Do not over fill the blender. Work in batches.
5. Return soup to the pan and add coconut milk, and season with salt and pepper. Heat before serving.

Tip: If coconut milk is not available, substitute 2% lowfat milk.

SALADS

Black Bean, Corn and Tomato Salad
Serves 4 (1 cup servings)

Ingredients:

1 can (15 oz.) black beans, drained and rinsed
½ cup frozen corn, thawed
2 plum tomatoes, seeded and chopped
¼ cup red onion, chopped
¼ cup cilantro, chopped
2 Tbsp vegetable oil
1 Tbsp lime juice (about 1 lime)

Directions:

1. In a large bowl, gently mix together beans, corn, tomatoes, onion and cilantro.
2. Add lime juice and oil. Stir to coat. Season with salt and pepper to taste.
3. Can be served immediately or set aside for 30 minutes for flavors to intensify.

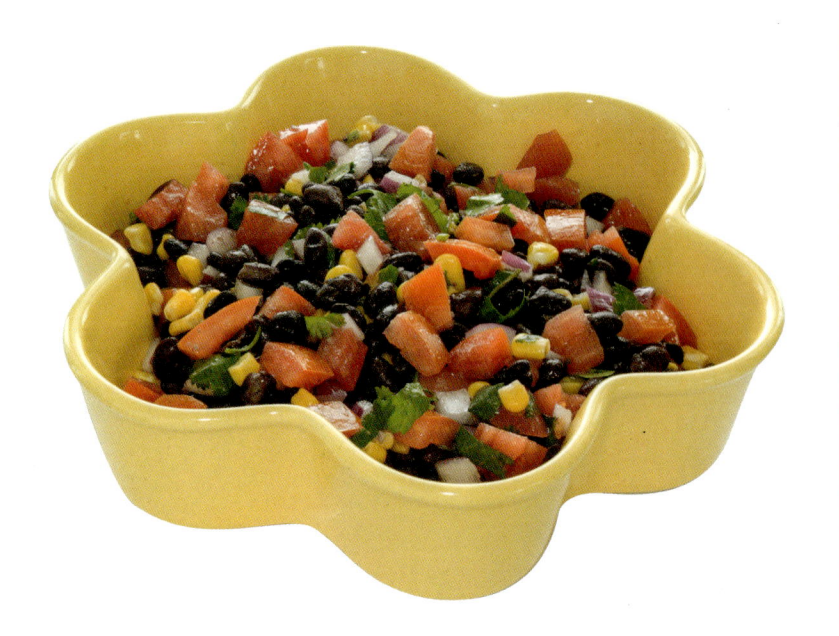

Nutrition Facts

4 servings per recipe

Serving size	1 cup

Amount Per Serving

Calories 450

	% Daily Value*
Total Fat 8g	10%
Saturated Fat 6g	30%
Trans Fat 0g	
Cholesterol 0mg	0%
Sodium 10mg	0%
Total Carbohydrate 73g	27%
Dietary Fiber 18g	64%
Total Sugars 4g	
Includes 0g Added Sugars	0%
Protein 24g	
Vitamin D 0mcg	0%
Calcium 140mg	10%
Iron 5.5mg	30%
Potassium 1630mg	35%

* The % Daily Value (DV) tells you how much a nutrient in a serving of food contributes to a daily diet. 2,000 calories a day is used for general nutrition advice.

Ramen Noodle Slaw
Serves 6 (1 cup servings)

Ingredients:

1 (14 oz.) bag coleslaw mix
4 green onions, chopped
¼ cup slivered almonds
½ cup raisins
1 (3-oz.) package ramen noodles, oriental flavor

Dressing:
⅓ cup vegetable oil
Ramen noodle seasoning packet
¼ cup cider vinegar
2 Tbsp sugar

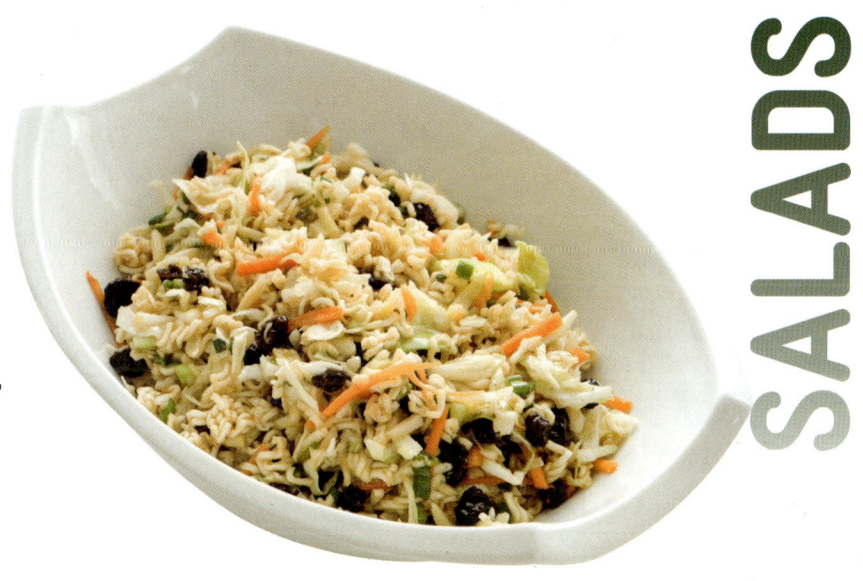

SALADS

Directions:
1. Crush ramen noodles into small pieces. Combine the coleslaw, green onions, almonds, raisins and ramen noodles in a salad bowl.
2. In a small bowl whisk the dressing ingredients. Pour the dressing over the slaw mixture and toss well.
3. Refrigerate for 2 hours before serving.

Nutrition Facts

6 servings per container

Serving size	1 cup

Amount Per Serving

Calories 250

	% Daily Value*
Total Fat 15g	19%
Saturated Fat 10g	50%
Trans Fat 0g	
Cholesterol 0mg	0%
Sodium 270mg	12%
Total Carbohydrate 26g	9%
Dietary Fiber 2g	7%
Total Sugars 14g	
Includes 4g Added Sugars	8%
Protein 3g	
Vitamin D 0mcg	0%
Calcium 40mg	2%
Iron 1.3mg	8%
Potassium 130mg	2%

* The % Daily Value (DV) tells you how much a nutrient in a serving of food contributes to a daily diet. 2,000 calories a day is used for general nutrition advice.

MYPLATE-STYLE TOSSED SALAD

Build a well-balanced tossed salad with foods from all five food groups!

1. Start with a bowl of salad greens.
2. Add chopped, diced and sliced vegetables, fruits, proteins, grains and dairy.
3. Toss with your favorite dressing.

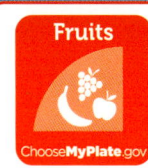

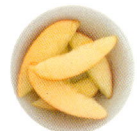

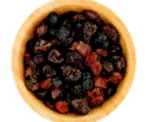

Fruits
ChooseMyPlate.gov

- Apples
- Dried Mixed Berries
- Orange Segments

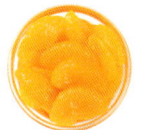

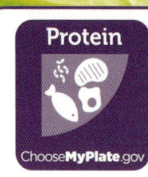

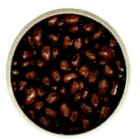

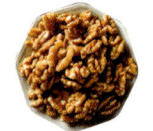

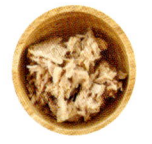

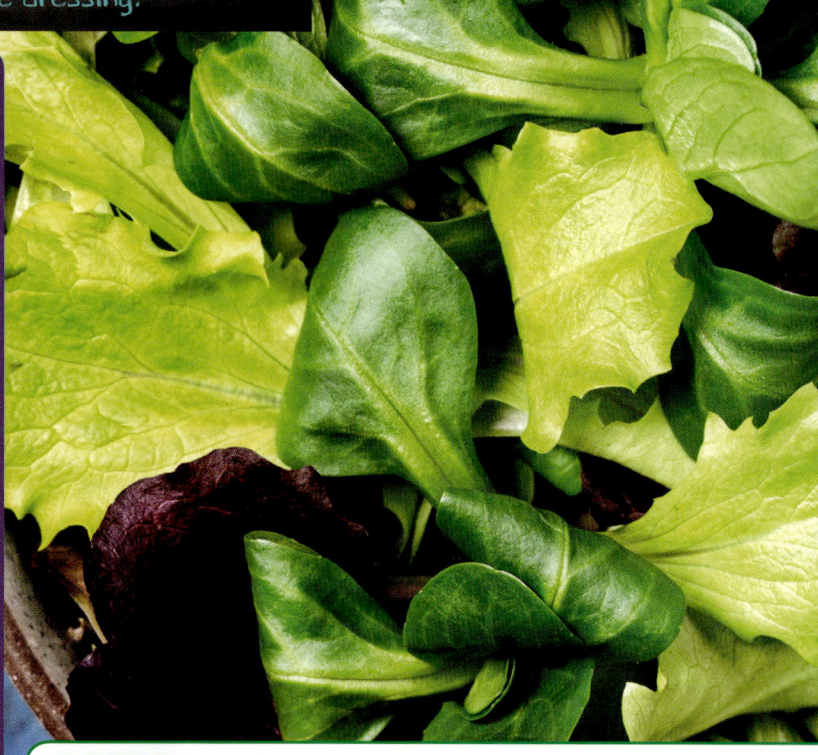

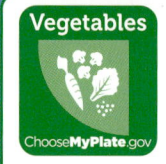

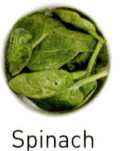

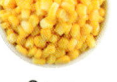

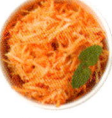

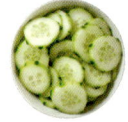

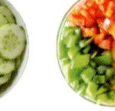

Protein
ChooseMyPlate.gov

- Beans
- Walnuts
- Canned Tuna

Vegetables
ChooseMyPlate.gov

- Spinach
- Corn
- Carrots
- Cucumbers
- Pep

Grains — ChooseMyPlate.gov
- Croutons
- Quinoa

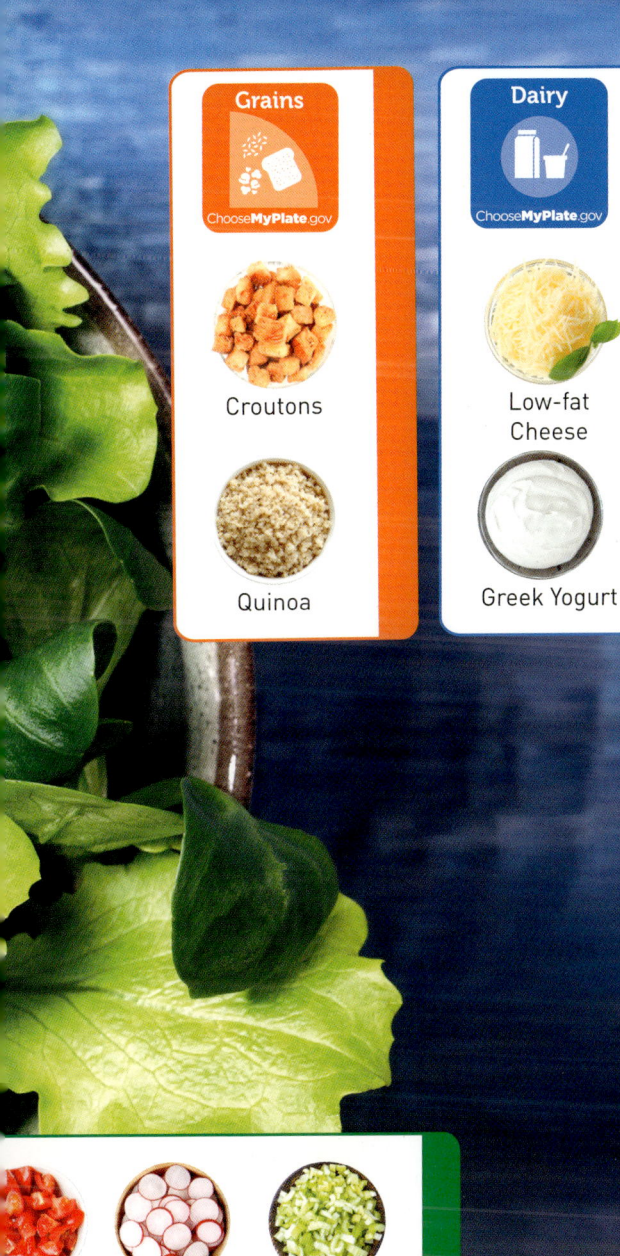

Dairy — ChooseMyPlate.gov
- Low-fat Cheese
- Greek Yogurt

Tomatoes · Radishes · Celery

HOMEMADE SALAD DRESSING
EASY AS 1-2-3

1. Use an airtight container with a tight-fitting lid.
2. Add ingredients from a recipe below.
3. Cover and shake!

IT'S THAT EASY!

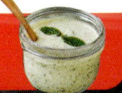

Classic French Dijon
- 3/4 cup vegetable oil
- 1/4 cup white wine vinegar
- 1/2 tsp dijon mustard

Creamy Dill
- 1/2 cup plain yogurt
- 1/2 cup mayonnaise
- 1 tsp lemon juice
- 1 Tbsp fresh dill, chopped

Honey Mustard
- 1/2 cup yellow mustard
- 1/4 cup honey
- 1/4 cup vegetable oil
- 1/2 Tbsp lemon juice

Each recipe makes about 1 cup, which is enough to dress several salads. Store leftover dressing in the fridge for up to 1 week.

SALADS

Carrot Pineapple Salad
Serves 3 (1 cup servings)

Ingredients:

2 cups shredded carrots (about 5 carrots)
1 can (8 oz.) crushed pineapple, drained

Dressing:
2 Tbsp plain yogurt
2 Tbsp lowfat mayonnaise
1 tsp sugar

Directions:
1. Combine carrots and pineapple in a bowl.
2. Mix yogurt and mayonnaise in a small bowl. Pour yogurt mixture over carrots and raisins and mix gently to coat the carrot mixture.
3. Chill until serving time.

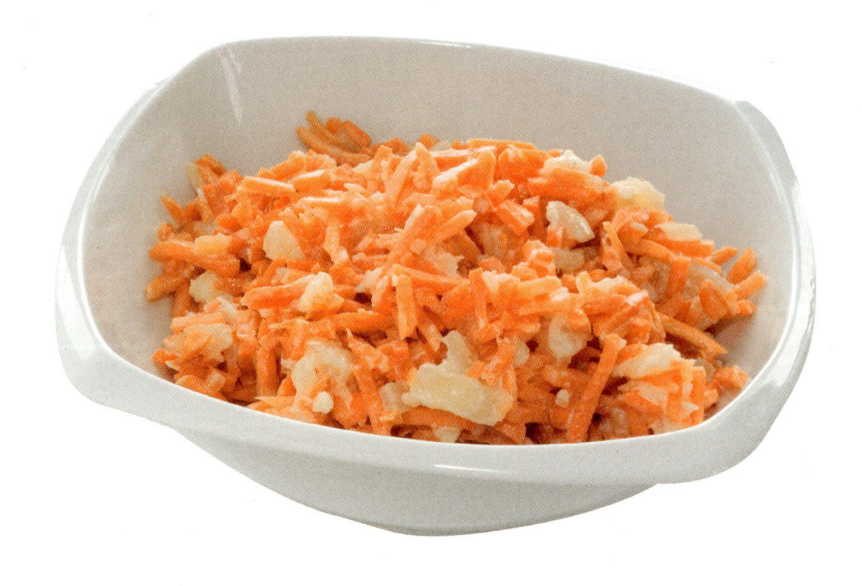

Nutrition Facts

3 servings per recipe

Serving size (1 cup)

Amount Per Serving

Calories 120

	% Daily Value*
Total Fat 2g	3%
Saturated Fat 0.5g	3%
Trans Fat 0g	
Cholesterol <5mg	1%
Sodium 85mg	4%
Total Carbohydrate 23g	8%
Dietary Fiber 3g	11%
Total Sugars 18g	
Includes 1g Added Sugars	2%
Protein 2g	
Vitamin D 0mcg	0%
Calcium 30mg	2%
Iron 0.6mg	4%
Potassium 110mg	2%

* The % Daily Value (DV) tells you how much a nutrient in a serving of food contributes to a daily diet. 2,000 calories a day is used for general nutrition advice.

Creamed Spinach Baked Potatoes
Serves 4

Ingredients:

4 Russet baking potatoes
1 tsp vegetable oil

Directions:
1. Preheat the oven to 425°F.
2. Scrub potatoes with water and pat dry.
3. Rub the potatoes with vegetable oil and poke them with a fork. Lay them directly on the oven rack.
4. Cook the potatoes for 45 to 60 minutes, until the skin is crispy.

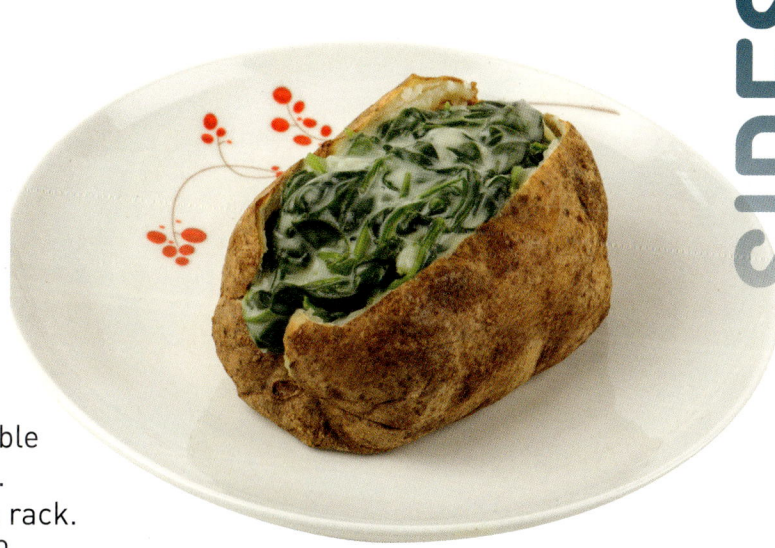

SIDES

Nutrition Facts

4 servings per recipe

Serving size	1/4 recipe

Amount Per Serving

Calories 340

	% Daily Value*
Total Fat 9g	12%
Saturated Fat 6g	30%
Trans Fat 0g	
Cholesterol 25mg	8%
Sodium 180mg	8%
Total Carbohydrate 53g	19%
Dietary Fiber 7g	25%
Total Sugars 9g	
Includes 0g Added Sugars	0%
Protein 12g	
Vitamin D 1mcg	6%
Calcium 270mg	20%
Iron 3.6mg	20%
Potassium 1370mg	30%

* The % Daily Value (DV) tells you how much a nutrient in a serving of food contributes to a daily diet. 2,000 calories a day is used for general nutrition advice.

Creamed Spinach Ingredients:

2 Tbsp butter
1 small onion, minced (about 1 cup)
3 Tbsp flour
1 ½ cups lowfat milk
1 bag (10 oz.) spinach, chopped

Directions:
1. In a large saucepan, cook minced onions in butter over medium heat until soft, about 5 minutes.
2. Sprinkle flour over the onion mixture, stir and cook the mixture for 2 minutes.
3. Add spinach and milk; cook 7-8 minutes until the mixture is thick and creamy.
4. Slice open a baked potato and add creamed spinach.

SIDES

Fried Rice-Style Quinoa
Serves 5 (1 cup servings)

Ingredients:

2 cups cooked quinoa
2 eggs
1 tsp butter
1 Tbsp vegetable oil
3 garlic cloves, minced
2 green onions, sliced
1 ½ cups frozen peas and carrots
¼ cup raisins
3 Tbsp soy sauce

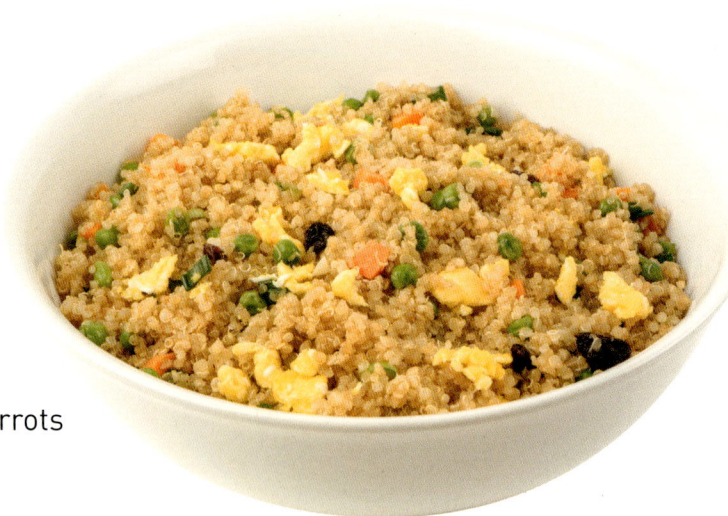

Directions:

1. Make 2 cups of quinoa according to package directions and set aside.
2. In a large non-stick skillet or wok, melt butter over medium heat. Break eggs into the butter and stir fry until dry. Remove the egg from the pan and set aside.
3. Add oil and garlic to the pan, cook over medium heat for 2 minutes. Add green onions, peas and carrots. Stir fry for about 3-4 minutes.
4. Add quinoa, egg, raisins and soy sauce. Stir-fry until heated through, about 3 minutes. Remove from heat and serve.

Nutrition Facts

5 servings per recipe

Serving size	**1 cup**

Amount Per Serving

Calories 200

	% Daily Value*
Total Fat 7g	9%
Saturated Fat 3.5g	18%
Trans Fat 0g	
Cholesterol 75mg	25%
Sodium 620mg	27%
Total Carbohydrate 29g	11%
Dietary Fiber 4g	14%
Total Sugars 8g	
Includes 0g Added Sugars	0%
Protein 8g	
Vitamin D 0mcg	0%
Calcium 50mg	4%
Iron 2.2mg	10%
Potassium 300mg	6%

* The % Daily Value (DV) tells you how much a nutrient in a serving of food contributes to a daily diet. 2,000 calories a day is used for general nutrition advice.

Candied Brussels Sprouts and Carrots — Serves 4

Ingredients:
16 brussels sprouts, trimmed and cut in half
24 baby carrots
2 Tbsp butter
2 Tbsp brown sugar

Directions:
Add 1 cup water, brussels sprouts and carrots to a saucepan. Bring to a boil. Turn heat down, cover and simmer 10 minutes. Drain off water. Return the pan of vegetables to the stove and add butter and brown sugar to the pan on low heat. Stir to coat the vegetables and melt the butter and brown sugar. Serve.

Nutrition Facts Servings: 4, **Serv. Size: 1 cup**, Amount Per Serving: **Calories 120**, **Total Fat** 6g (8% DV), Sat. Fat 3.5g (18% DV), Trans Fat 0g, **Cholest.** 15mg (5% DV), **Sodium** 100mg (4% DV), **Total Carb.** 17g (6% DV), Fiber 4g (14% DV), Total Sugars 10g (Incl. 7g Added Sugars, 14% DV), **Protein** 3g, Vit. D (0% DV), Calcium (4% DV), Iron (8% DV), Potas. (8% DV).

Green Beans, Corn and Bacon — Serves 4

Ingredients:
2 strips bacon
1 ear sweet corn, kernels cut off cob
1 Tbsp butter
¾ pound (12-oz.) green beans, washed and trimmed

Directions:
Slice bacon into small (½-inch) pieces and fry in saucepan until crispy. Remove the bacon from pan and drain on paper towel. Set aside. Leave 1 Tbsp of bacon grease in the pan and add the corn kernels. Cook about 5 minutes over medium high heat. Place beans in microwave-safe dish, cover and cook on HIGH for 3-4 minutes. Toss with butter and place in serving dish. Spoon the corn mixture over the green beans and sprinkle with bacon bits. Serve.

Nutrition Facts Servings: 4, **Serv. Size: 1 cup**, Amount Per Serving: **Calories 110**, **Total Fat** 8g (10% DV), Sat. Fat 4g (20% DV), Trans Fat 0g, **Cholest.** 25mg (8% DV), **Sodium** 85mg (4% DV), **Total Carb.** 8g (3% DV), Fiber 2g (7% DV), Total Sugars 2g (Incl. 0g Added Sugars, 0% DV), **Protein** 3g, Vit. D (0% DV), Calcium (2% DV), Iron (4% DV), Potas. (4% DV).

SIDES

Stir and Serve Mushrooms — Serves 4

Ingredients:

8 oz. mushrooms, cleaned and cut in half
2 Tbsp margarine
1 garlic clove, minced
1 tsp soy sauce

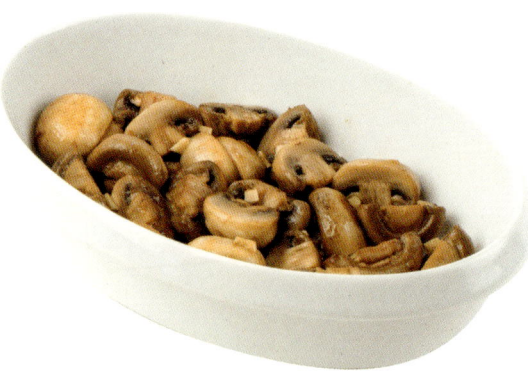

Directions:

In a large skillet melt margarine over medium heat. Add mushrooms, stirring constantly over medium heat for 2 minutes. Stir in garlic and soy sauce and cook for another 2 minutes. Serve.

Nutrition Facts Servings: 4, **Serv. Size: 1/4 recipe**, Amount Per Serving: **Calories 60**, **Total Fat** 6g (8% DV), **Sat. Fat** 1g (5% DV), Trans Fat 1g, **Cholest.** 0mg (0% DV), **Sodium** 130mg (6% DV), **Total Carb.** <1g (0% DV), Fiber 0g (0% DV), Total Sugars 0g (Incl. 0g Added Sugars, 0% DV), **Protein** 1g, Vit. D (0% DV), Calcium (0% DV), Iron (0% DV), Potas. (2% DV).

Kale Chips — Serves 4

Ingredients:

1 head kale
2 Tbsp vegetable oil
¼ tsp salt

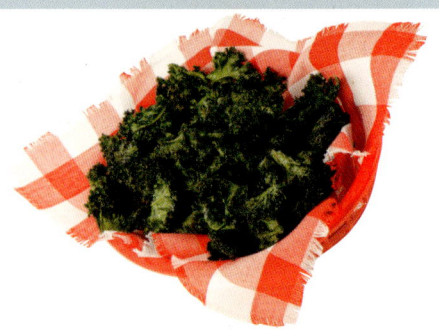

Directions:

Preheat oven to 300°F. Rinse and dry kale. Remove the center ribs and stems from each leaf. Tear the leaves into 3-4-inch pieces. In a large bowl toss kale with olive oil using your hands to rub each piece of kale with the oil. Spread kale in single layer on 2 baking sheets lined with foil. Lightly sprinkle the kale with salt. Bake for 18-20 minutes. Remove from oven. Store in an air-tight container for up to 1 week.

Nutrition Facts Servings: 4, **Serv. Size: 1/4 recipe**, Amount Per Serving: **Calories 90**, **Total Fat** 7g (9% DV), **Sat. Fat** 6g (30% DV), Trans Fat 0g, **Cholest.** 0mg (0% DV), **Sodium** 170mg (7% DV), **Total Carb.** 6g (2% DV), Fiber 2g (7% DV), Total Sugars 2g (Incl. 0g Added Sugars, 0% DV), **Protein** 3g, Vit. D (0% DV), Calcium (8% DV), Iron (6% DV), Potas. (8% DV).

Avocado Hummus

Serves 6 (¼ cup servings)

Ingredients:
1 can (15 oz.) chickpeas (garbanzo beans), rinsed and drained
1 avocado, pit and skin removed
1 garlic clove, peeled and chopped
2 Tbsp smooth peanut butter
2 Tbsp vegetable oil
2 Tbsp lemon juice (about 1 lemon)
¼ cup water

Directions:
Place all the ingredients in a blender and process until smooth. If needed, add 1-2 Tbsp more water for a creamy texture.

A tasty spread on sandwiches.

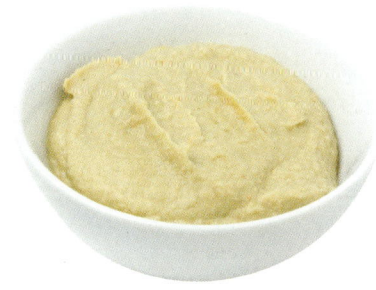

Nutrition Facts Servings: 6, Serv. Size: 1/6, Amount Per Serving: **Calories 230**, **Total Fat** 14g (18% DV), Sat. Fat 5g (25% DV), Trans Fat 0g, **Cholest.** 0mg (0% DV), **Sodium** 200mg (9% DV), **Total Carb.** 22g (8% DV), Fiber 8g (29% DV), Total Sugars 5g (Incl. 0g Added Sugars, 0% DV), **Protein** 7g, Vit. D (0% DV), Calcium (4% DV), Iron (6% DV), Potas. (6% DV).

Corn Relish

Serves 6 (¼ cup servings)

Ingredients:
1 ½ cups fresh or frozen corn
1 Tbsp vegetable oil
¼ cup cilantro, chopped
2 Tbsp red onion, minced
2 tsp apple cider vinegar
1 tsp sugar
½ tsp cumin

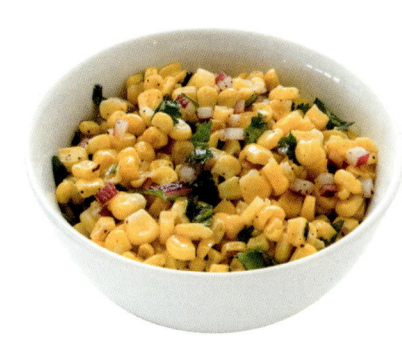

Great with hot dogs and hamburgers.

Directions:
Cook corn in the oil over medium-high heat for 3 minutes. Pour corn into a bowl and let cool a few minutes. Add the rest of the ingredients to the bowl and toss gently to combine.

Nutrition Facts Servings: 6, **Serv. Size: 1/6**, Amount Per Serving: **Calories 50**, **Total Fat** 2.5g (3% DV), Sat. Fat 2g (10% DV), Trans Fat 0g, **Cholest.** 0mg (0% DV), **Sodium** 0mg (0% DV), **Total Carb.** 8g (3% DV), Fiber <1g (3% DV), Total Sugars 2g (Incl. <1g Added Sugars, 1% DV), **Protein** 1g, Vit. D (0% DV), Calcium (0% DV), Iron (2% DV), Potas. (2% DV).

SALSAS, SAUCES & DIPS

SALSAS, SAUCES & DIPS

Cucumber Yogurt Sauce
Serves 6 (¼ cup servings)

Ingredients:
¾ cup plain yogurt
1 cucumber, peeled
¼ tsp garlic powder
1 Tbsp fresh lemon juice

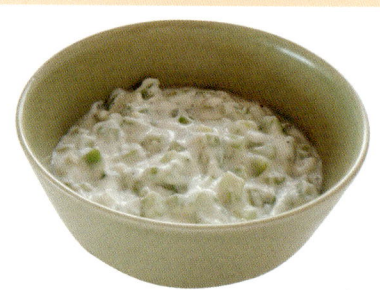

Directions:
Cut cucumber in half, scoop out seeds with a spoon. Dice cucumber, place in a paper towel and squeeze gently to remove water. In a medium bowl, gently stir the yogurt, cucumber, garlic powder and lemon juice.

Serve with grilled chicken, lamb or turkey burgers.

Nutrition Facts Servings: 6, **Serv. Size: 1/6,** Amount Per Serving: **Calories 25, Total Fat** 1g (1% DV), Sat. Fat 0.5g (3% DV), Trans Fat 0g, **Cholest.** <5mg (1% DV), **Sodium** 20mg (1% DV), **Total Carb.** 3g (1% DV), Fiber 0g (0% DV), Total Sugars 2g (Incl. 0g Added Sugars, 0% DV), **Protein** 1g, Vit. D (2% DV), Calcium (4% DV), Iron (0% DV), Potas. (2% DV).

Fresh Tomato Salsa
Serves 6 (¼ cup servings)

Ingredients:
1 ½ cups (about 3) plum/roma tomatoes
2 Tbsp red onion, diced
2 Tbsp cilantro, chopped
1 jalapeño pepper, seeded and minced
1 Tbsp lime juice
1 Tbsp vegetable oil

Directions:
Cut tomatoes in half and squeeze them to remove the seeds. Discard seeds and dice the tomatoes. Gently mix all ingredients in a bowl.

Delicious with scrambled eggs.

Nutrition Facts Servings: 6, **Serv. Size: 1/6,** Amount Per Serving: **Calories 35, Total Fat** 2.5g (3% DV), Sat. Fat 2g (10% DV), Trans Fat 0g, **Cholest.** 0mg (0% DV), **Sodium** 0mg (0% DV), **Total Carb.** 4g (1% DV), Fiber <1g (2% DV), Total Sugars 2g (Incl. 0g Added Sugars, 0% DV), **Protein** 1g, Vit. D (0% DV), Calcium (4% DV), Iron (4% DV), Potas. (0% DV).

Pan Roasted Chicken and Vegetables
Serves 4

Ingredients:

8 red potatoes, washed and cut into 1-inch chunks
½ large onion, cut into 1-inch pieces
20 baby carrots
1 package (8 oz.) mushrooms
4 (1½ pounds) bone-in chicken thighs, skin removed

Roasting Seasoning:
3 Tbsp vegetable oil
3 garlic cloves, minced
1 tsp salt
1½ tsp dried rosemary, crushed
¾ tsp pepper
½ tsp paprika

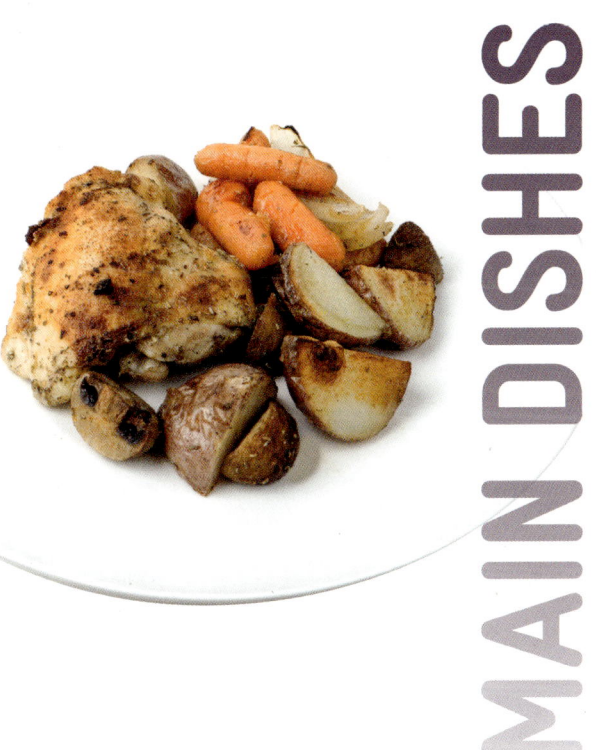

MAIN DISHES

Directions:
1. Preheat oven to 425°F. Spray 9X13-inch baking pan with cooking spray.
2. In small bowl, whisk the roasting seasoning ingredients together.
3. In a large bowl, combine potatoes, onions, mushrooms and carrots. Pour half of the roasting seasoning over the vegetables and toss to coat evenly. Spread vegetables in a single layer in the baking pan.
4. Place the chicken in the bowl with the rest of the roasting seasoning. Toss to coat and place the chicken pieces over vegetables.
5. Roast the vegetables and chicken in the oven until a thermometer inserted in chicken reads 170°F-175°F and vegetables are just tender, 40-45 minutes.
6. Remove from oven and serve.

Nutrition Facts
4 servings per recipe
Serving size 1/4 recipe

Amount Per Serving
Calories 470

	% Daily Value*
Total Fat 13g	17%
Saturated Fat 9g	45%
Trans Fat 0g	
Cholesterol 35mg	12%
Sodium 720mg	31%
Total Carbohydrate 75g	27%
Dietary Fiber 9g	32%
Total Sugars 8g	
Includes 0g Added Sugars	0%
Protein 17g	
Vitamin D 0.1mcg	0%
Calcium 80mg	6%
Iron 4.3mg	25%
Potassium 2200mg	45%

* The % Daily Value (DV) tells you how much a nutrient in a serving of food contributes to a daily diet. 2,000 calories a day is used for general nutrition advice.

MAIN DISHES

Sweet Potato Burritos with Avocado Crema
Serves 6

Ingredients:

2 sweet potatoes, peeled and diced
½ cup (4 oz.) store-bought salsa
2 Tbsp cilantro, chopped
2 Tbsp vegetable oil
½ small onion, diced
1 cup canned black beans, rinsed and drained
1 ½ cups pepper jack cheese, shredded
6 (8-inch) flour tortillas
Avocado Crema (recipe below)

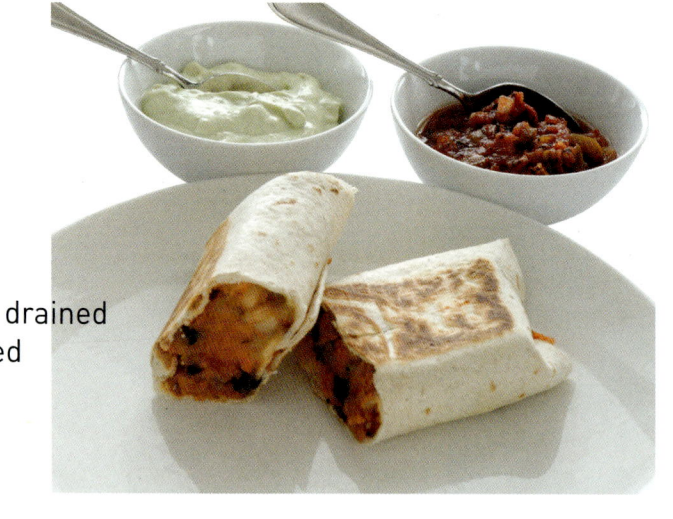

Directions:

1. Place sweet potatoes in a pot and cover with water. Cover pot with a lid and bring to a boil. Turn heat down to low and simmer for 15 minutes. Drain water. Mash sweet potatoes with a fork or potato masher. Stir in salsa and cilantro.
2. Heat oil in a skillet pan over medium heat, add onions, and cook for 5 minutes. Add beans to the onion mixture. Cook for 2 more minutes. Turn off heat. Stir in sweet potato mixture.
3. To make each burrito, spoon ¾ cup of the filling and ¼ cup shredded cheese on to a tortilla and roll up the tortillas. Repeat this step 5 more times to make 6 burritos.
4. Brown two sides of each burrito in a non-stick pan over medium heat.
5. Serve with avocado crema.

Avocado Crema: Mash 1 pitted avocado with ¼ cup sour cream and 1 Tbsp lime juice in a bowl.

Nutrition Facts

6 servings per recipe
Serving size: 1 burrito

Amount Per Serving
Calories 440

	% Daily Value*
Total Fat 22g	28%
Saturated Fat 11g	55%
Trans Fat 0g	
Cholesterol 35mg	12%
Sodium 790mg	34%
Total Carbohydrate 48g	17%
Dietary Fiber 9g	32%
Total Sugars 7g	
Includes 0g Added Sugars	0%
Protein 16g	
Vitamin D 0mcg	0%
Calcium 320mg	25%
Iron 2.9mg	15%
Potassium 580mg	10%

* The % Daily Value (DV) tells you how much a nutrient in a serving of food contributes to a daily diet. 2,000 calories a day is used for general nutrition advice.

Zucchini Lasagna
Serves 4

Ingredients:

4 zucchinis (each about 7" long)
2 cups (16 oz.) pasta sauce
1 cup part-skim ricotta cheese
½ cup grated parmesan cheese
1½ cups part-skim mozzarella cheese, shredded
½ tsp Italian seasoning
¼ tsp garlic powder

Directions:
1. Heat oven to 375°F. Lightly spray 9X9-inch baking dish with cooking spray.
2. Spread ½ cup tomato sauce in bottom of baking dish; set aside.
3. In medium bowl, stir together the ricotta cheese, parmesan cheese, ½ cup shredded mozzarella cheese, Italian seasoning and garlic powder.
4. Cut the zucchini into ¼ inch slices long wise. Place zucchini slices on a paper towel and then on a microwave-safe plate. Put the plate in the microwave and cook on HIGH for 4 minutes.
5. Remove the zucchini slices from the microwave. Let cool 5 minutes. Pat dry with the paper towel.
6. With ⅓ of the zucchini strips, line the bottom of the pan. Spoon one-half of the ricotta filling onto each of the zucchini slices. Repeat this step two times, changing the direction of zucchini strips for each step.
7. Spread the remaining tomato sauce evenly over the top and sprinkle with shredded mozzarella cheese.
8. Bake about 25 minutes or until golden and bubbly. Let stand 10 minutes before serving.

MAIN DISHES

Nutrition Facts

4 servings per recipe
Serving size 1/4 recipe

Amount Per Serving
Calories 330

	% Daily Value*
Total Fat 19g	24%
Saturated Fat 10g	50%
Trans Fat 0.5g	
Cholesterol 55mg	18%
Sodium 1070mg	47%
Total Carbohydrate 16g	6%
Dietary Fiber 3g	11%
Total Sugars 8g	
Includes 4g Added Sugars	8%
Protein 25g	
Vitamin D 0.3mcg	2%
Calcium 650mg	50%
Iron 1.6mg	10%
Potassium 620mg	15%

* The % Daily Value (DV) tells you how much a nutrient in a serving of food contributes to a daily diet. 2,000 calories a day is used for general nutrition advice.

MAIN DISHES

Creamy Pasta Primavera
Serves 4

Ingredients:

8 oz. spiral (rotini) dried pasta
1 cup asparagus, trimmed and cut in 2-inch pieces
½ cup red pepper, diced
1 small yellow summer squash, cut into thin circles
5 baby carrots, cut into thin strips
2 Tbsp vegetable oil
4 oz. cream cheese, cubed
½ cup parmesan cheese, grated
2 Tbsp lemon juice

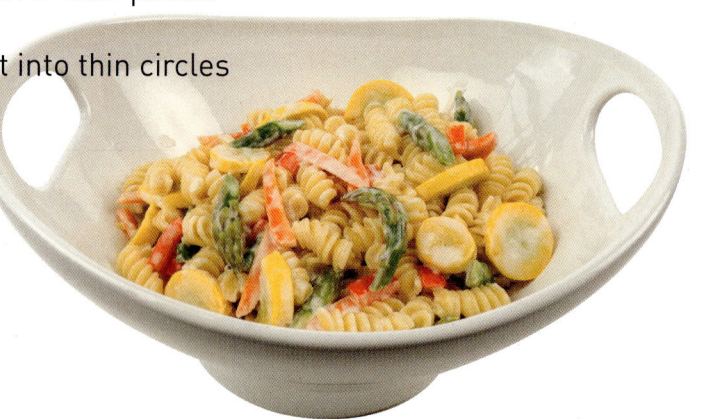

Directions:

1. Cook the pasta according to package directions. Add the asparagus, bell peppers, zucchini and carrots to the boiling water for the last 3 minutes of cooking. Pour ½ cup of pasta water into a measuring cup. Drain the pasta and vegetables into a strainer or colander.
2. In the same pot used for the pasta, add the pasta water, cream cheese, parmesan cheese and lemon juice. Stir until the cheese is melted. Add the pasta and vegetables, and gently toss with sauce.

Tip: Using flavored cream cheese, such as garlic herb, instead of plain cream cheese, will add additional flavor to this dish.

Nutrition Facts

4 servings per recipe
Serving size: 1/4 recipe

Amount Per Serving
Calories 440

	% Daily Value*
Total Fat 22g	28%
Saturated Fat 13g	65%
Trans Fat 0g	
Cholesterol 40mg	13%
Sodium 310mg	13%
Total Carbohydrate 51g	19%
Dietary Fiber 8g	29%
Total Sugars 5g	
Includes 0g Added Sugars	0%
Protein 15g	
Vitamin D 0.2mcg	2%
Calcium 290mg	20%
Iron 3.9mg	20%
Potassium 190mg	4%

* The % Daily Value (DV) tells you how much a nutrient in a serving of food contributes to a daily diet. 2,000 calories a day is used for general nutrition advice.

The Storytellers

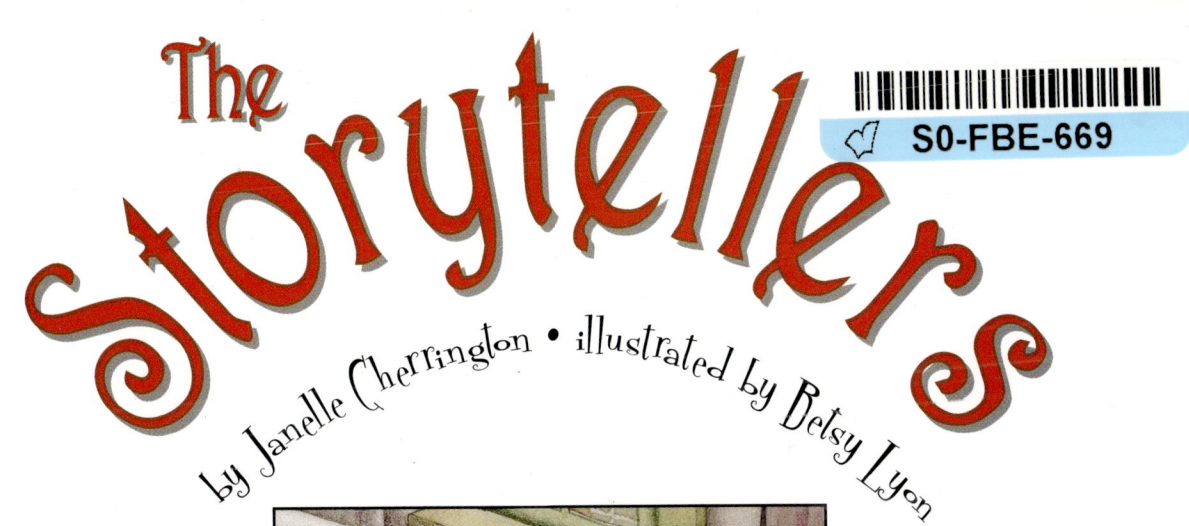

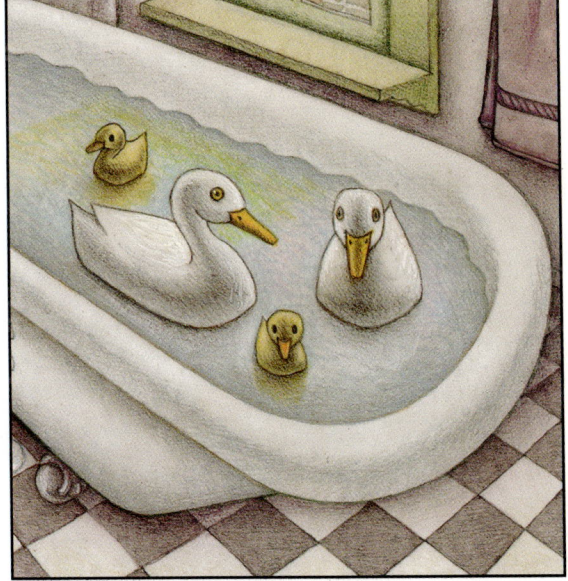

by Janelle Cherrington • illustrated by Betsy Lyon

SCHOLASTIC INC.
New York   Toronto   London   Auckland   Sydney
Mexico City   New Delhi   Hong Kong   Buenos Aires

No part of this publication may be reproduced in whole or in part, or stored in a retrieval system, or transmitted in any form or by any means, electronic, mechanical, photocopying, recording, or otherwise, without written permission of the publisher. For information regarding permission, write to Scholastic Inc., Education Group, 555 Broadway, New York, NY 10012.

Developed by Kirchoff/Wohlberg, Inc., in cooperation with Scholastic Inc.
Credits appear on the inside back cover, which constitutes an extension of this copyright page.
Copyright © 2002 by Scholastic Inc.
All rights reserved.   Published by Scholastic Inc.   Printed in the U.S.A.
ISBN 0-439-35134-0
SCHOLASTIC and associated logos and designs are trademarks
and/or registered trademarks of Scholastic Inc.

3 4 5 6 7 8 9 10   23   09 08 07 06 05

Hi!

Think of your favorite book. Did you ever ask yourself, "How did the writer think of this story?"

Think of a book with beautiful pictures. Did you ever wonder how the artist knew what to draw?

You are about to meet some famous authors and illustrators. You'll learn about the work they do. They go through many steps to write stories or make pictures.

Are you ready? Let's get started!

Robert McCloskey

At first, Robert McCloskey wanted to be the kind of artist whose pictures are in museums. He made paintings filled with fancy creatures from his imagination. Nobody bought his paintings, though. Then an editor that he knew gave him some good advice. The editor told Robert McCloskey that he should create pictures of ordinary things from his own life.

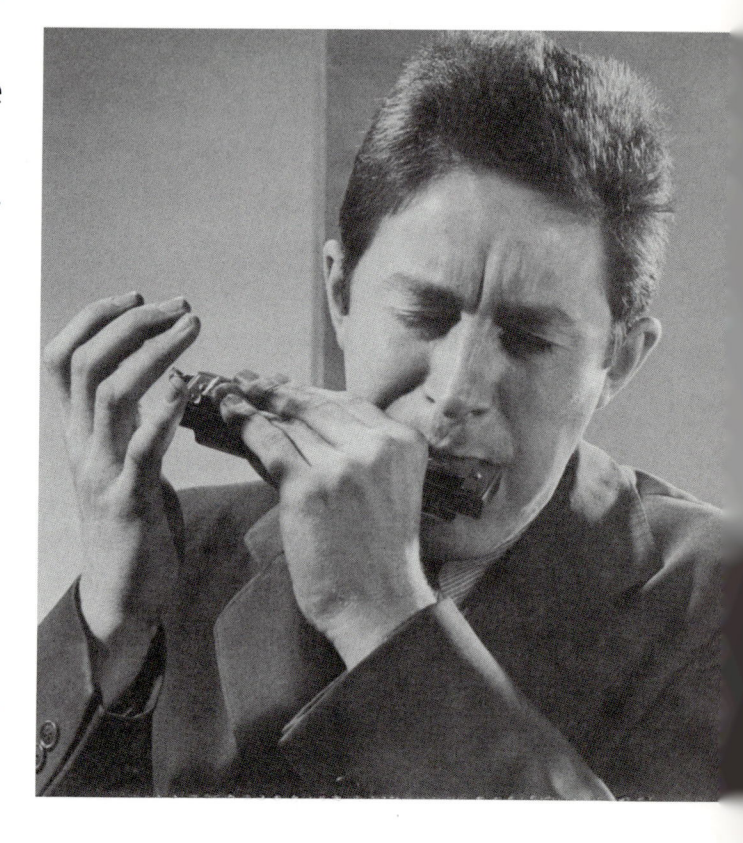

MAKE WAY FOR DUCKLINGS

Robert McCloskey

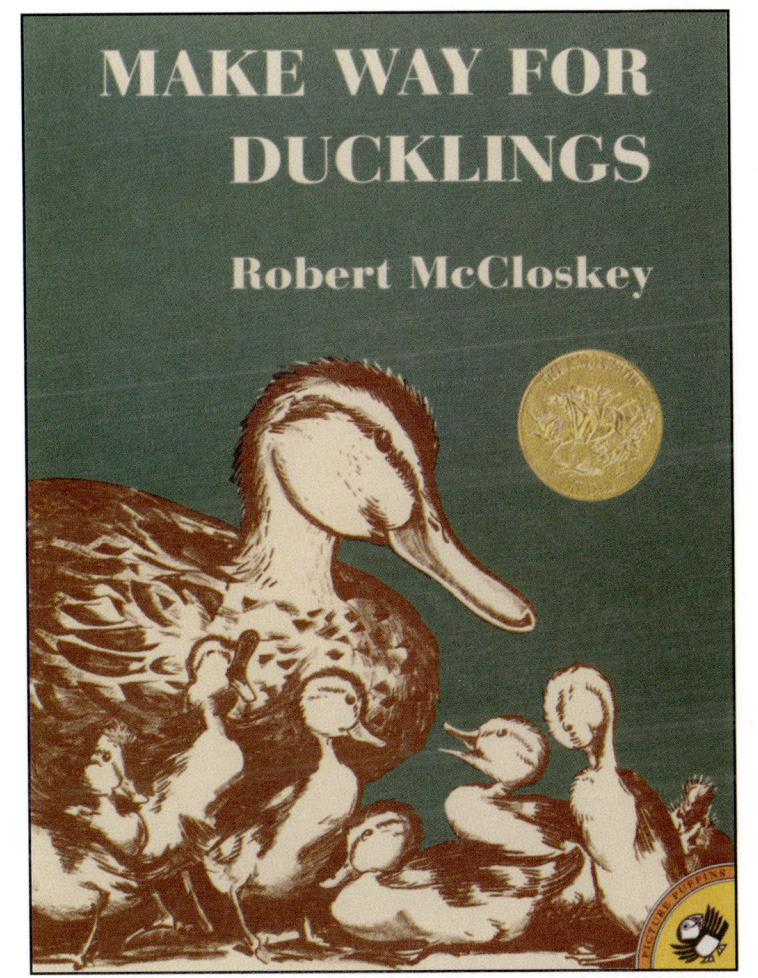

From MAKE WAY FOR DUCKLINGS by Robert McCloskey, copyright 1941, renewed ©1969 by Robert McCloskey. Used by permission of Viking Penguin, an imprint of Penguin Putnam Books for Young Readers, a division of Penguin Putnam Inc.

How do you draw a duck that really looks like a duck? Robert McCloskey asked himself that question when he was drawing the pictures for his famous book, *Make Way for Ducklings*.

What was his answer? It was "You more or less have to think like a duck!"

He thought the best way to think like a duck was to get to know some ducks. So that's what he did.

McCloskey began by making sketches. Sketches are practice drawings. When an artist likes the sketches, it is time to make the final painting or drawing. When all the final paintings are done, they are sent to an editor at a publishing company.

Robert McCloskey wanted his artwork to look just right. If he did not like a sketch, he would rip it up and start over. Sometimes he would do 20 or 30 sketches before he made a painting.

McCloskey did not like his sketches of ducklings at first. What do you think he did? He bought four live ducks. He took them to his New York City apartment!

McCloskey believed you have to know something to draw it well. He spent the next few weeks on his hands and knees. He followed the ducks around his apartment. He carried his sketchbook and his pen with him. He even watched them swim in his bathtub.

McCloskey says this helped him think like a duck. Soon, he drew pictures he liked. *Make Way for Ducklings* was born. Children still love it.

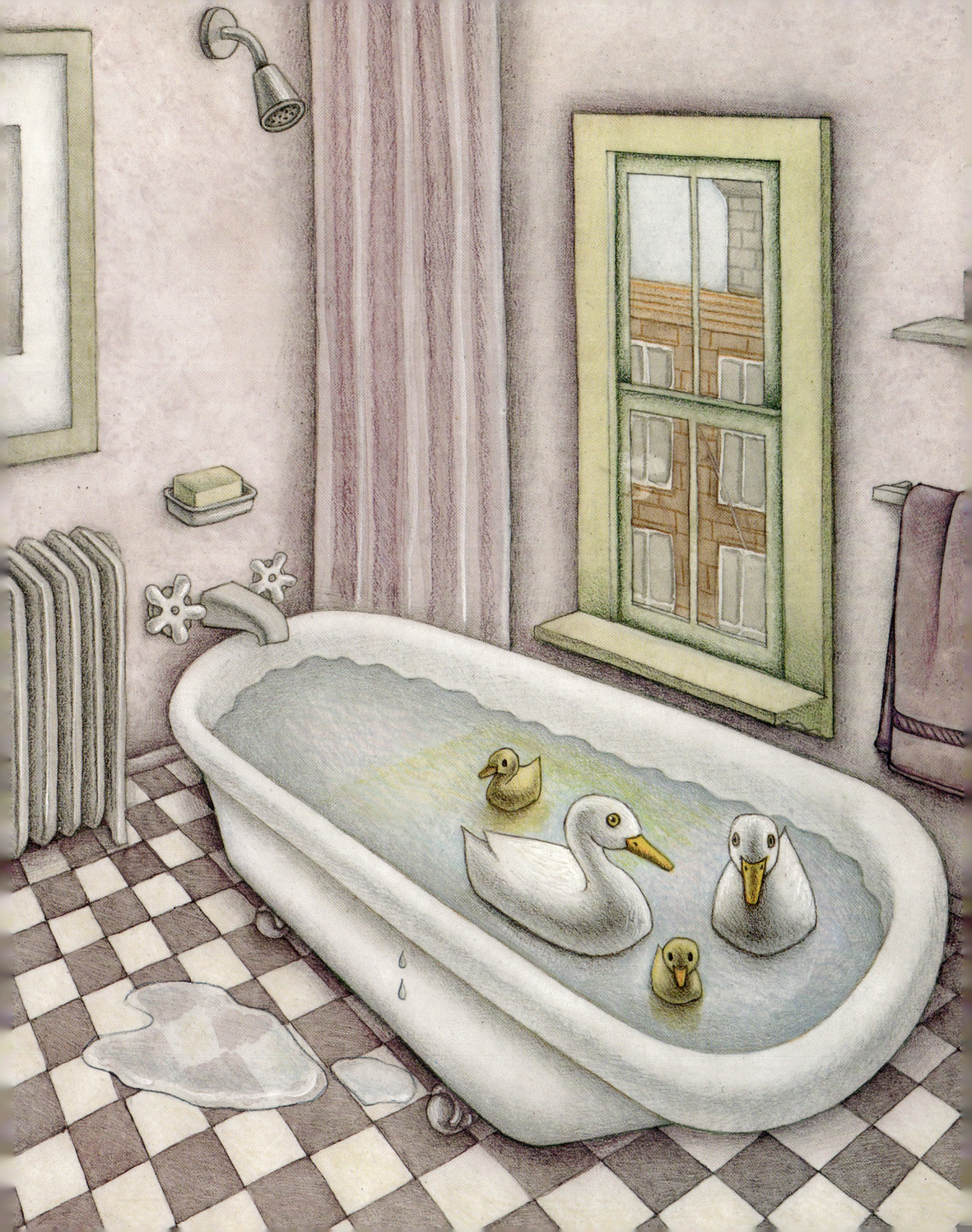

Virginia Hamilton

For Virginia Hamilton, writing is a lot like painting a picture. Pictures come to her mind when she writes. Then she tries to make those pictures with words. She wants her audience, her readers, to see what she sees.

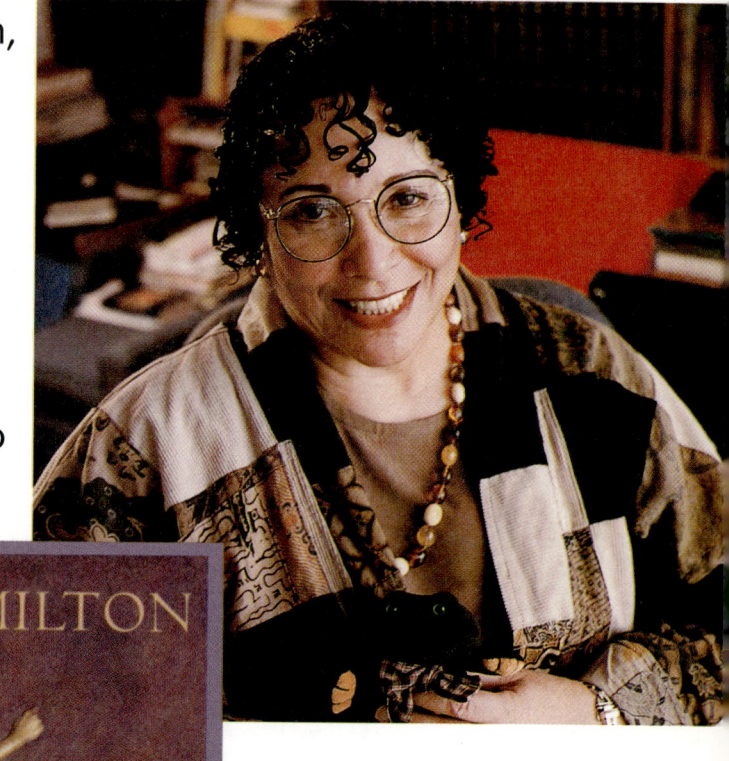

One time, she got a very clear picture in her head. She saw a boy running through the woods. Virginia ran after him in her mind. That boy became the main character of *M. C. Higgins, the Great*. The book won a famous prize!

M.C. Higgins, the Great is a book of fiction. The story, however, seems very real.

M.C. Higgins, the Great is about a boy who lives in the Ohio hills with his family. Strip mining has turned the area around the family home into a slag heap. As time goes on, the family home is threatened by the approaching strip mining process. The owners of the mines want to dig wherever they choose. M.C. wants his family to leave the area. He thinks leaving will get his family away from danger and improve their lives. However, the place has been home to the family for several generations. M.C. comes to learn how much the home means to them all and, with help from two strangers, decides that they must stay and fight to save what is theirs.

Virginia Hamilton has been writing books for over 30 years. She says she writes because she loves a good story. She also loves to see characters rise up out of nowhere.

Hamilton writes a lot about her childhood in Ohio. She has good memories of being young. She says she writes about three things. She writes about what she knows. She writes about what she remembers. She writes about what she imagines. These three subjects are her tools.

When Hamilton writes nonfiction, she starts by doing research. Hamilton looks for everything she can find about her subject. She finds books, diaries, letters, newspaper articles, magazine articles, and any other kind of information around. She does not stop looking until she is sure she is an expert on her subject.

She says you have to know as much about your subject as you know about yourself. Have you ever found out that much about something?

Once she finds the facts she needs, Virginia starts writing. She thinks nonfiction stories are not easy to write. She says it's hard to make all the facts come to life. It's hard to remember them all, too!

Some of her nonfiction books have to do with the historical struggle of African Americans against slavery. One of these books is *Anthony Burns: The Defeat and Triumph of a Fugitive Slave*. Virginia Hamilton said that she tried to write about a "true spirit, a gentle human being" who inspired others with his brave fight for freedom. The character, Anthony Burns, has those traits. Virginia Hamilton writes about him as though she knew and admired him. She makes readers feel that they know him and admire him too.

Anthony Burns is a boy who was born into slavery in Virginia. In 1854, at the age of twenty, he escaped and traveled north to Boston, where he lived and worked as a free man for a few months. However, a law of that time, called the Fugitive Slave Act, permitted a slave owner to follow and reclaim a runaway slave. Burns's former owner followed him to Boston and tried to take him back. The hearings in Boston caused riots and demonstrations as the two sides battled.

Virginia Hamilton believes children who want to become writers should write every day. She also thinks that good writers should read as much as they can. She says reading stirs up your imagination. What do you think she means?

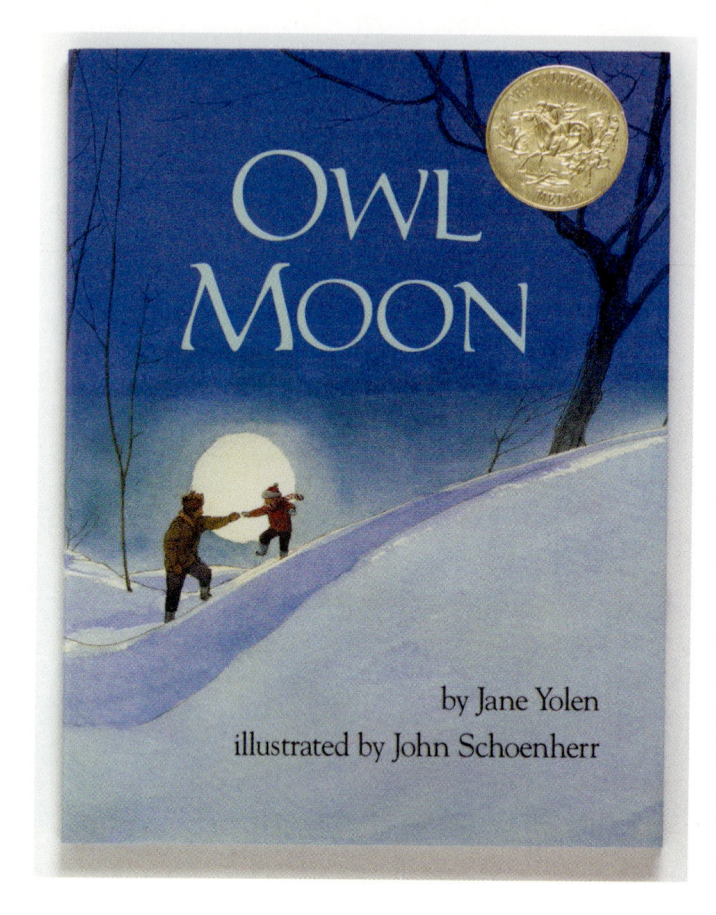

From OWL MOON by Jane Yolen, illustrated by John Schoenherr. ©1988 by John Schoenherr. Used by permission of Philomel Books, an imprint of Penguin Putnam Books for Young Readers, a division of Penguin Putnam Inc.

Jane Yolen

Jane Yolen has been writing since she was a child. She said her first writing experience was in first grade. She wrote a script for her class musical. The musical was about talking vegetables. Jane played the chief carrot. The big, final episode contained a singing salad!

When Jane Yolen was young, she read many folktales and sang many folk songs. These stories and songs still give her ideas for her own books.

Characters often pop into Jane Yolen's head, too. One time, someone asked Jane if she knows how a book is going to end as she writes it. She said that she often doesn't.

She says she keeps on writing because she wants to know what will happen to her characters. Once, when she was writing a book, she added a group of elves to the story. She didn't know where they came from!

She kept the elves out of her imagination for three weeks. Then, one day, she figured out why they were there. So they stayed.

Owl Moon is a book Jane Yolen wrote that is about waiting for something to happen. In this book, a girl and her father go out on a winter's night hoping to see a Great Horned Owl. It is very cold as they walk through the woods. Even though she is cold, the girl knows that she must be quiet and patient. The owl will not appear if there is any noise. At the same time, she knows that, even if she is patient and quiet, she still may not get to see an owl. The long search and wait ends happily, however. Jane Yolen's hard work had a happy result as well. Her book won an important prize.

Jane Yolen thinks of ideas for new stories all the time. What does she do with them? She keeps an idea file!

Jane Yolen says that ideas come "from all over." She gets them from paintings, other books, newspaper articles, dreams, even listening to other people's conversations! She also reads a lot. She likes to read all kinds of books, such as history books, poetry, fantasy novels, and mysteries.

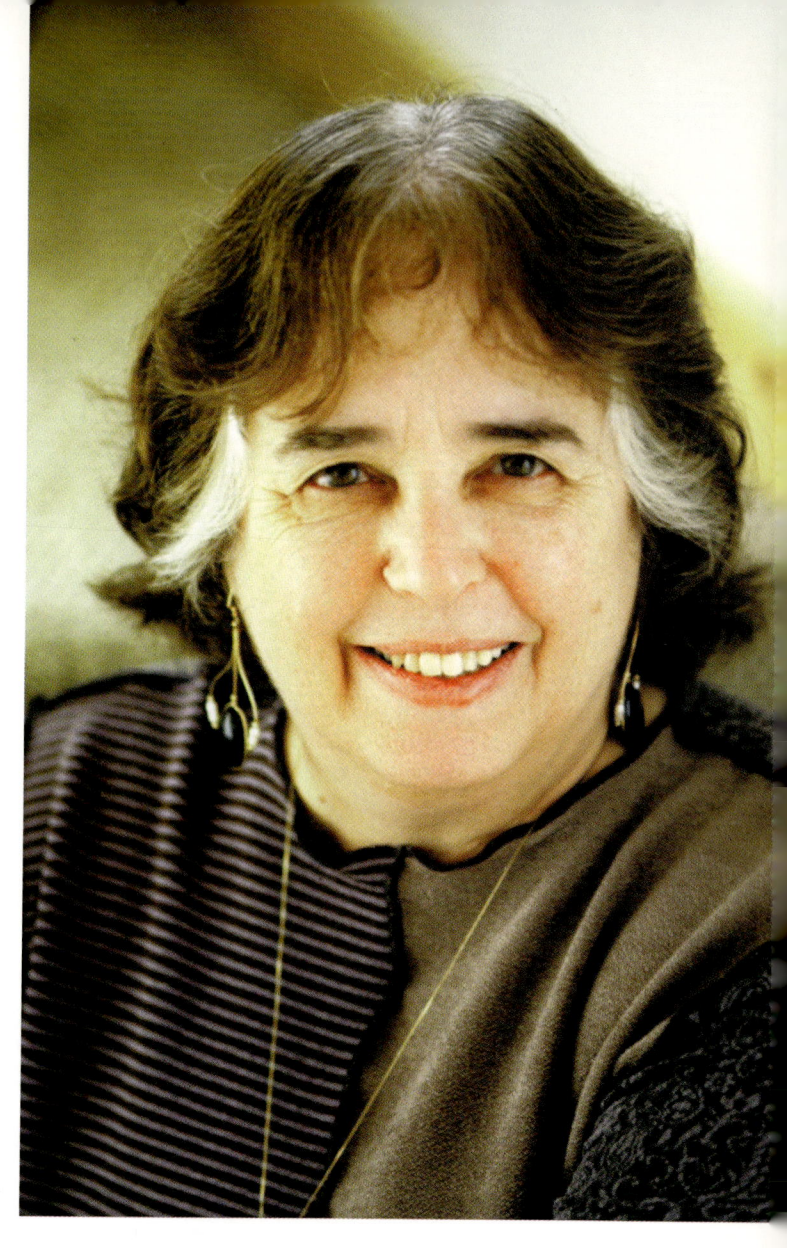

When Jane gets an idea, she writes it down. Then she puts the idea in a folder. She puts the folder in a file cabinet. Once in a while, she pulls out an idea she likes. She may work on it for a while. Most of Jane Yolen's ideas do not become books overnight. Some ideas take many years to turn into books.

Jane Yolen says that she sometimes starts her books this way. First, she thinks of a situation. Then she asks herself, what should happen next? The answer she gives to her question is the story she writes down.

Both of Jane Yolen's parents were writers. Her father wrote for the newspapers and her mother wrote short stories. Jane Yolen grew up surrounded by words. Jane Yolen became a journalist and poet before she started writing children's books.

Two of her books are songbooks for children. She says that most of the songs are those she heard as a child. Her father played the ukulele and guitar and her mother played the piano. They both sang the songs that Jane Yolen put in her books. She taught them to her own children and then in her books to an endless number of children. In Jane Yolen's Old MacDonald Songbook she quoted an old nursery rhyme as an invitation to read:

"Then let us sing merrily,
   merrily now,
We'll live on the custards
   that come from the cow."

Allen Say

Allen Say is an artist. He moved to Portland, Oregon in 1999. He has moved 37 times in his life.

Say's mother was born in America, but she moved to Japan as a teenager. His Korean father grew up in China with British foster parents. Say's mother and father married in Osaka, Japan. When Allen was young, he was sent to live with his grandmother in Tokyo.

Say makes pictures of the many different cultures he has seen.

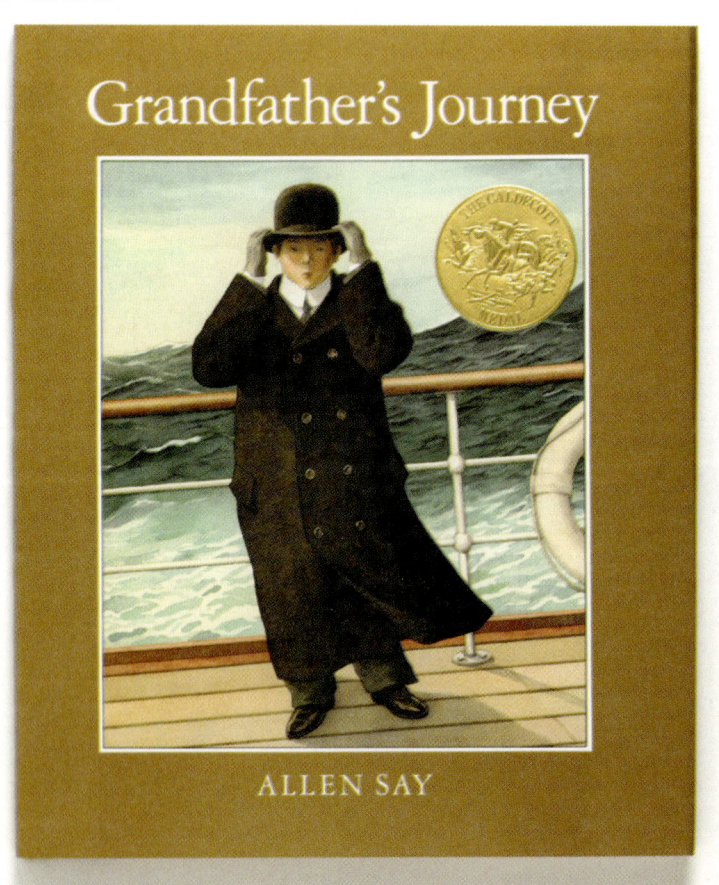

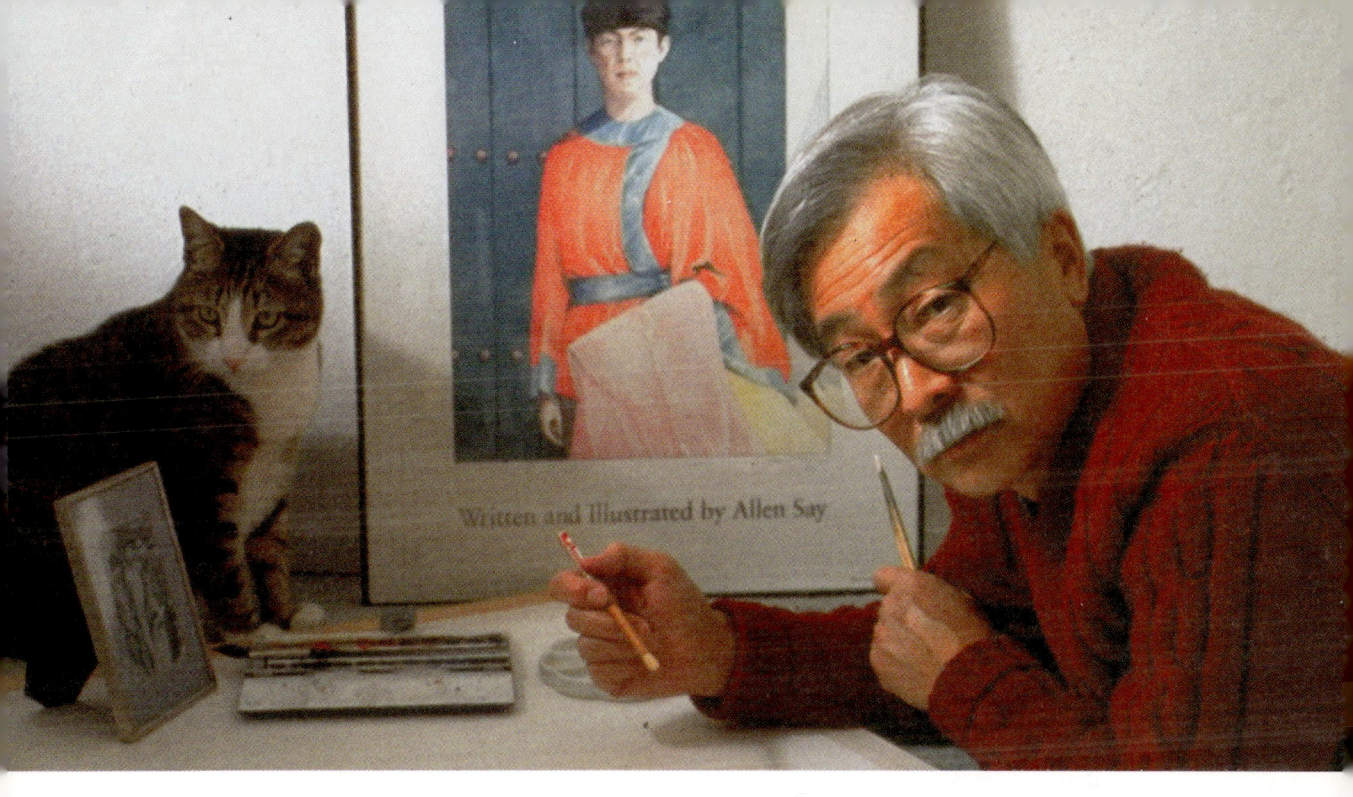

Allen Say always loved to draw. He says he started drawing before he could walk. He drew on everything. He even drew on walls! Say's father was not sure he wanted his son to be an artist. He thought his son should be a businessman. The boy kept drawing, anyway. He knew that he was good at creating beautiful pictures.

While Allen Say was still a young boy, he introduced himself to a famous cartoonist named Noro Shinpei. Shinpei liked him and let him do chores around the art studio. Soon Allen Say was helping Shinpei draw his art boards. Shinpei taught him, "to draw is to discover."

Allen Say worked with Shinpei until he was 15. Then the young artist moved to America.

Allen Say paints with watercolors. He is known for his precise style and for showing his characters in unexpected ways. For example, his book *El Chino* is about a Chinese American who decided to become a bullfighter. It was based on a true story. It is not often you see an Asian character dressed in a bullfighter's colorful Spanish outfit!

Say worked for an advertising company for many years. Once in a while, he illustrated children's stories. It wasn't until he was 50 that he found out he could also write stories.

One of the books that Allen Say illustrated and wrote was *Grandfather's Journey*. It is mostly about his grandfather's trip from Japan to America, but it is also about Allen Say's own experiences. Both grandson and grandfather become torn by strong feelings of affection and connection for both countries.

When he begins a new book, Say says he draws many sketches. Then he does a storyboard or picture map. This diagram shows how the book will be built. Next he starts painting. He writes the words last, in one or two days.

Do you think pictures tell stories? Look at a picture. Then try to write a story about it. Did you enjoy yourself? Maybe you can become an artist or a storyteller some day.

Leo
the Lion Cub

Story by Beverley Randell
Illustrations by Julian Bruère

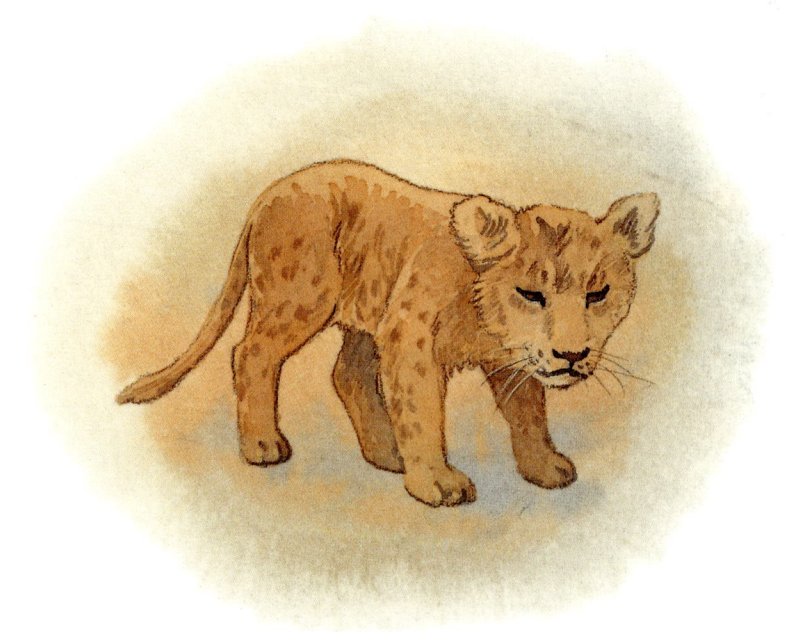

Leo belonged to a large family of lions,
called a pride.
When he was only six weeks old,
his mother died,
so his aunts took care of him.

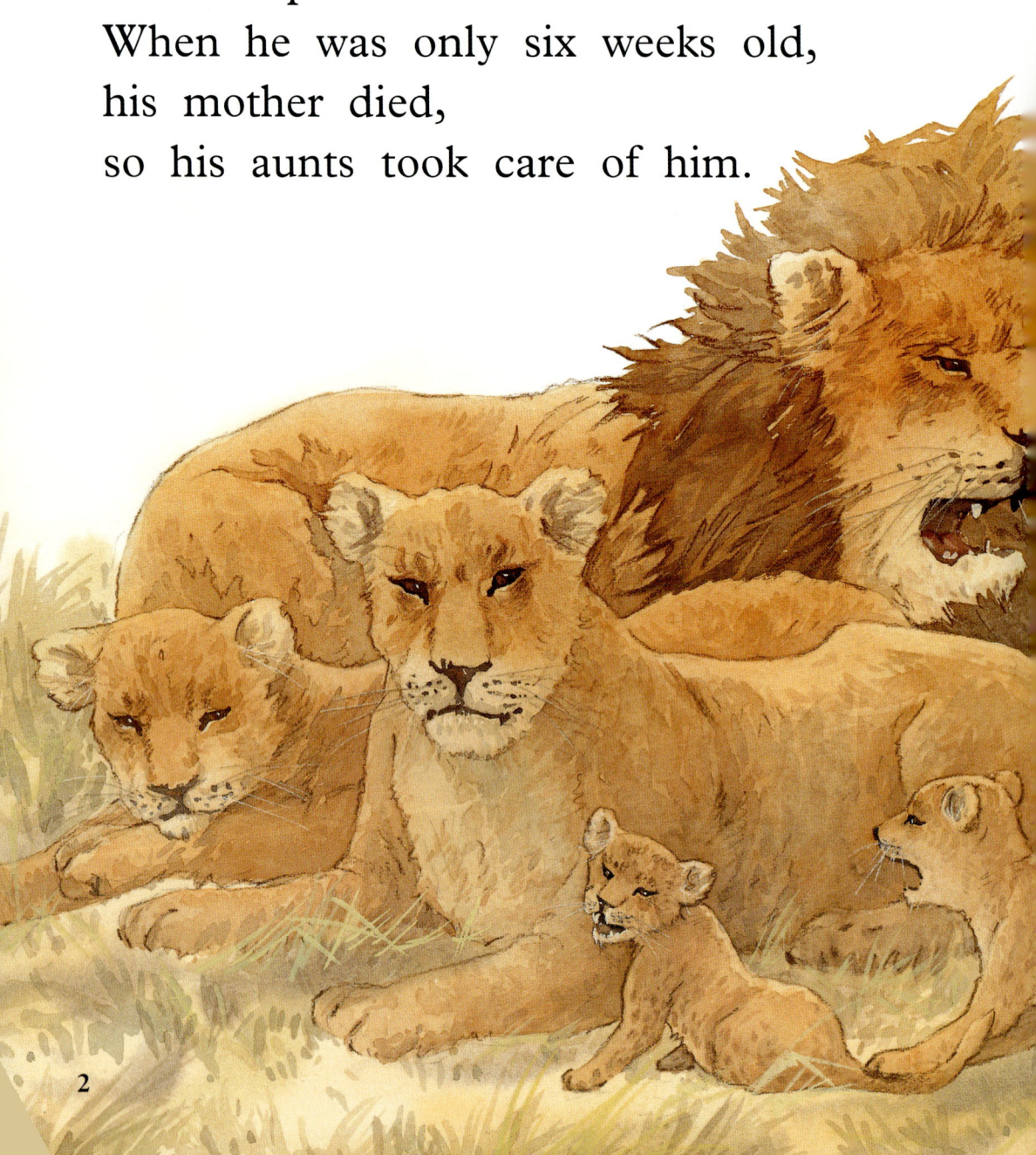

Leo was the youngest
and smallest cub in the pride.
All of his cousins were bigger
than he was.
They often knocked him over
when they played with him.
They liked pouncing on his tail
and biting it.

Leo had to be brave.
He had to learn how to fight.

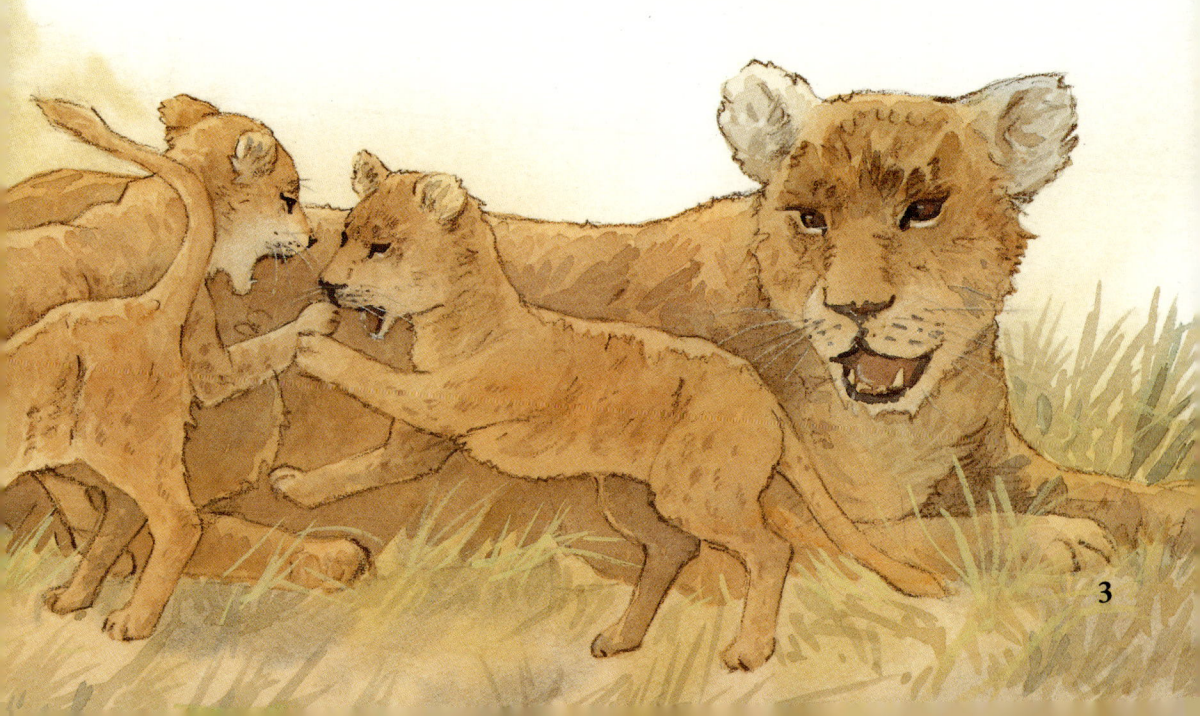

Soon it was time
for the pride to move on.
The lions needed to find
a new hunting ground.

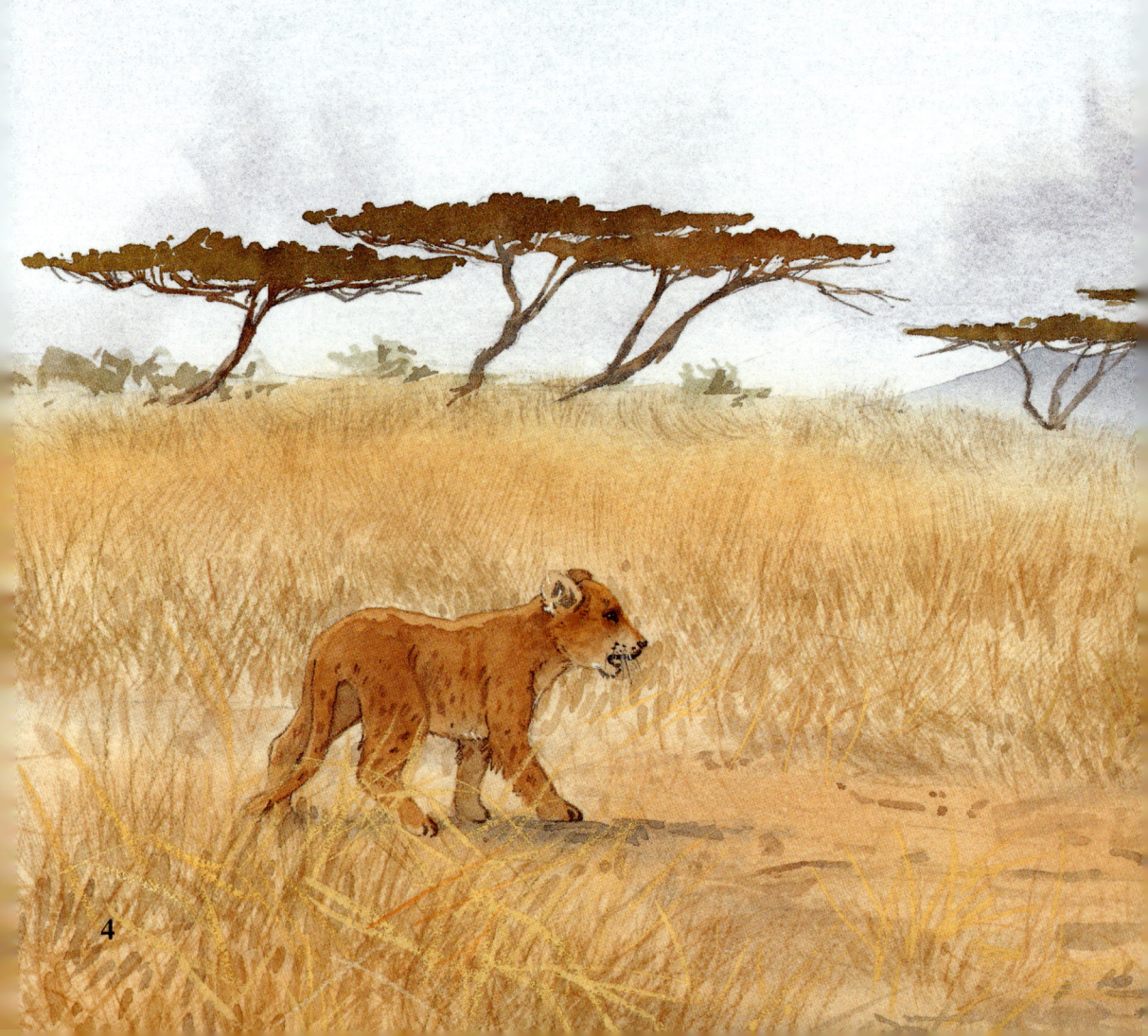

They padded off
through the dry grass,
one after the other.

But Leo could not keep up.
His little legs were too short.

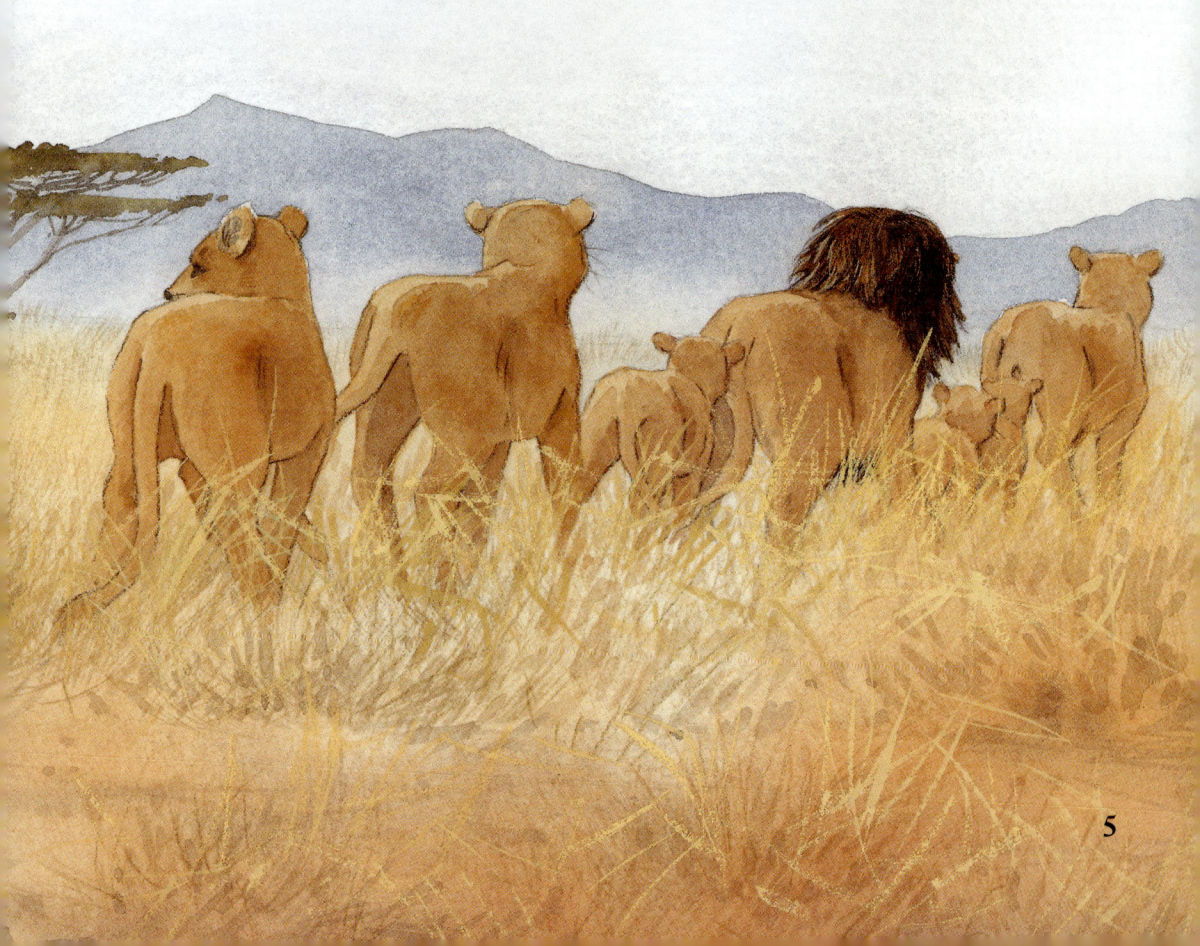

When Leo whimpered,
one of his aunts stopped.
He tried to catch up with her,
but he could not walk fast enough.
So she moved on without him.

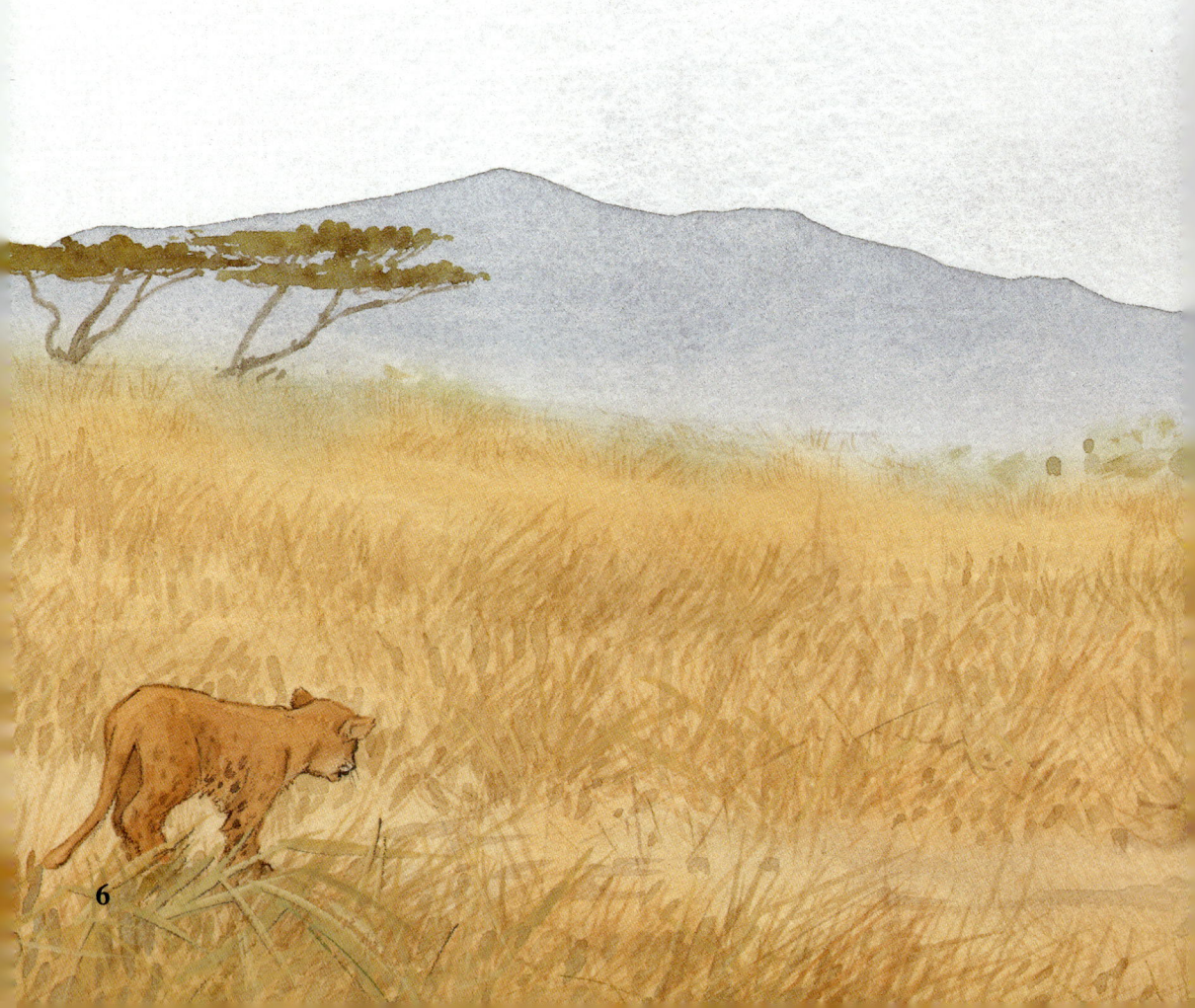

He was soon left behind.
He had never been alone before,
and he was afraid.

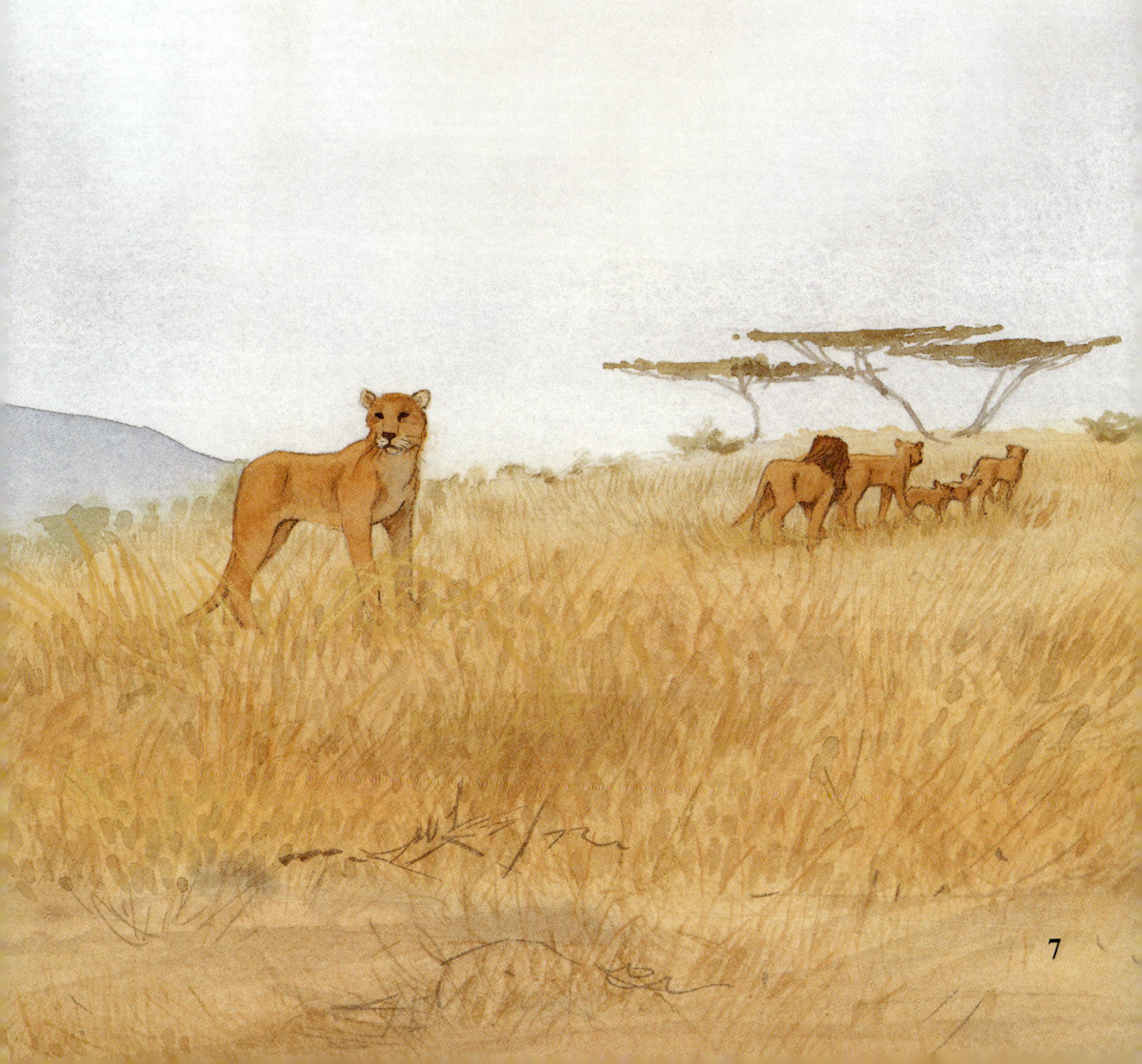

When the sun went down,
the night was full
of strange noises.

Leo heard some hyenas
howling in the distance.

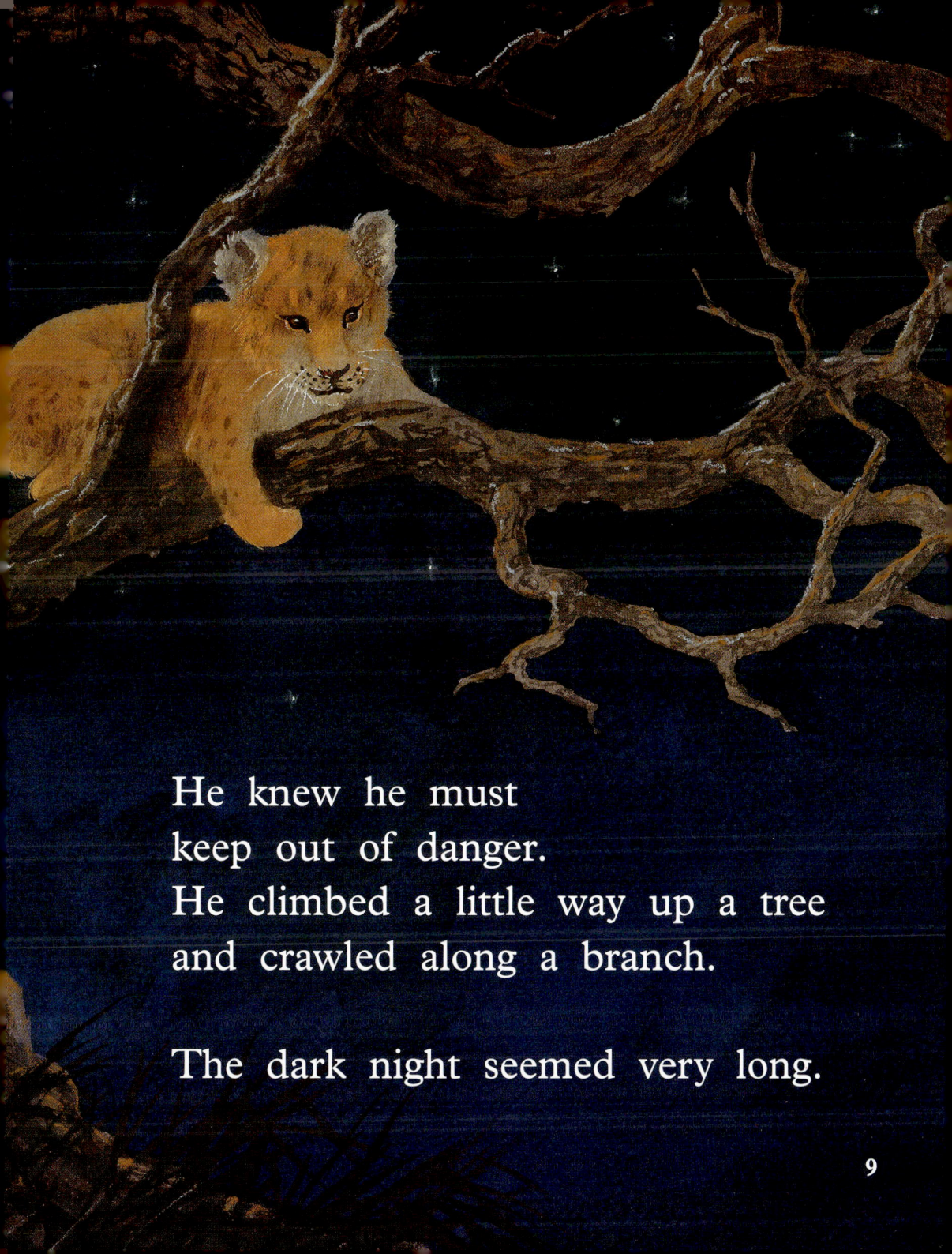

He knew he must
keep out of danger.
He climbed a little way up a tree
and crawled along a branch.

The dark night seemed very long.

The next day, Leo saw a lioness
walking through the long grass!
But when he ran to join her,
he found that he did not know her.
This lioness was a stranger
who growled fiercely at him.

Leo could see her huge jaws
and her sharp teeth.
He was terrified.

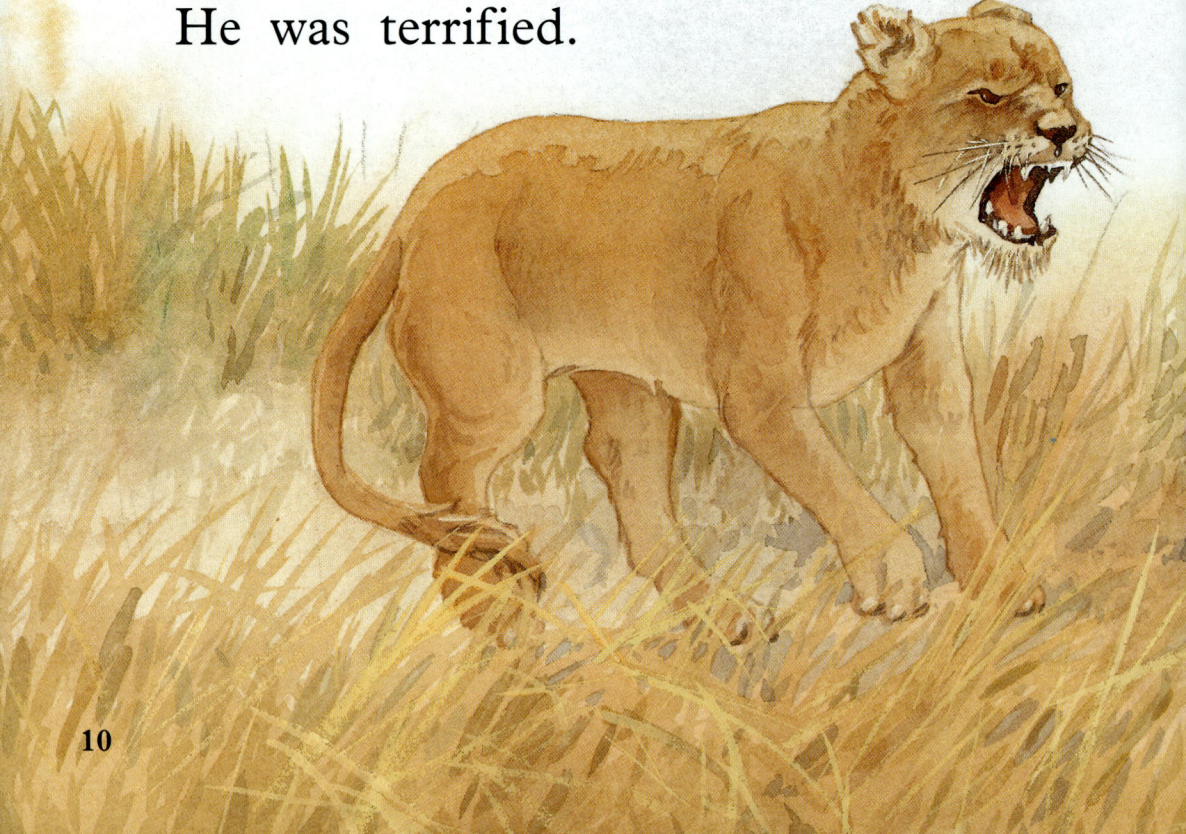

Instead of trying to run away,
Leo rolled onto his back.
That was his way of saying,
Don't hurt me!
I'm only a small cub!

Leo was lucky.
The lioness turned away
and left him alone.

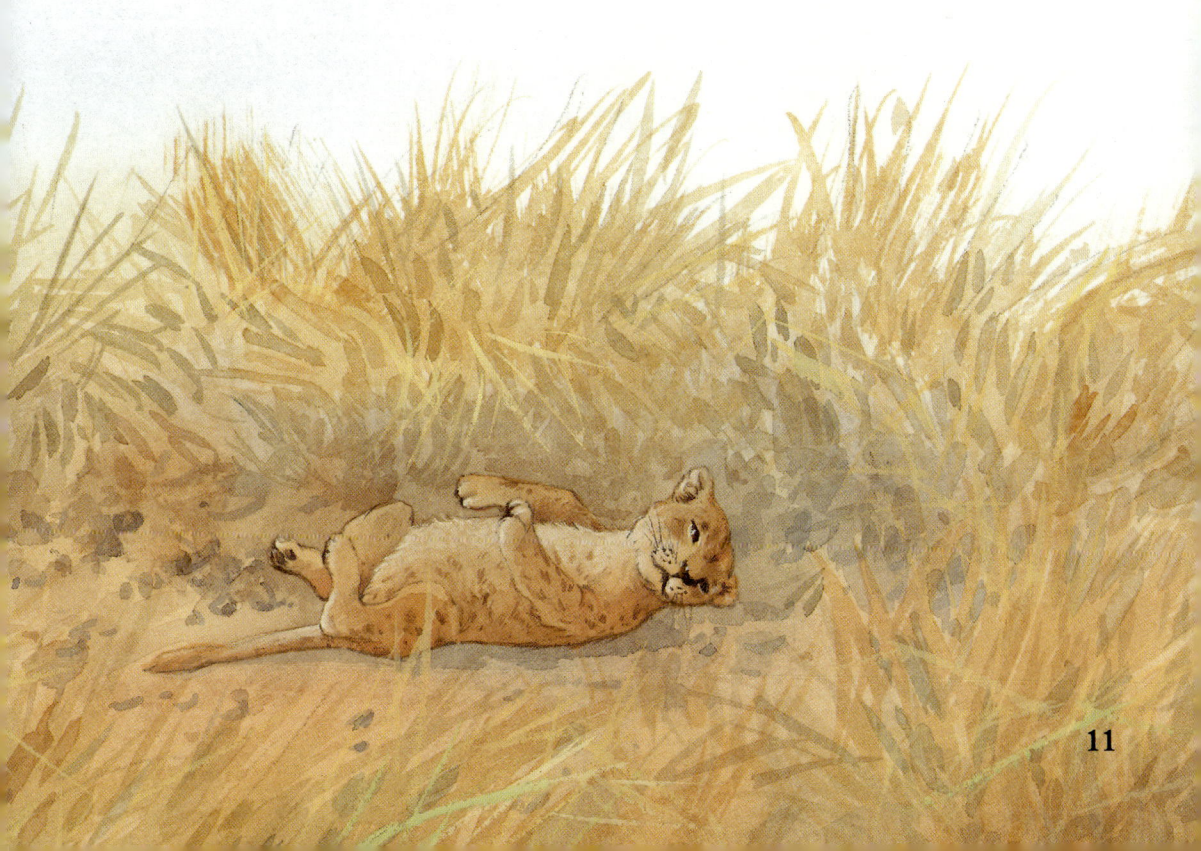

Leo had to spend
a second lonely night in a tree.

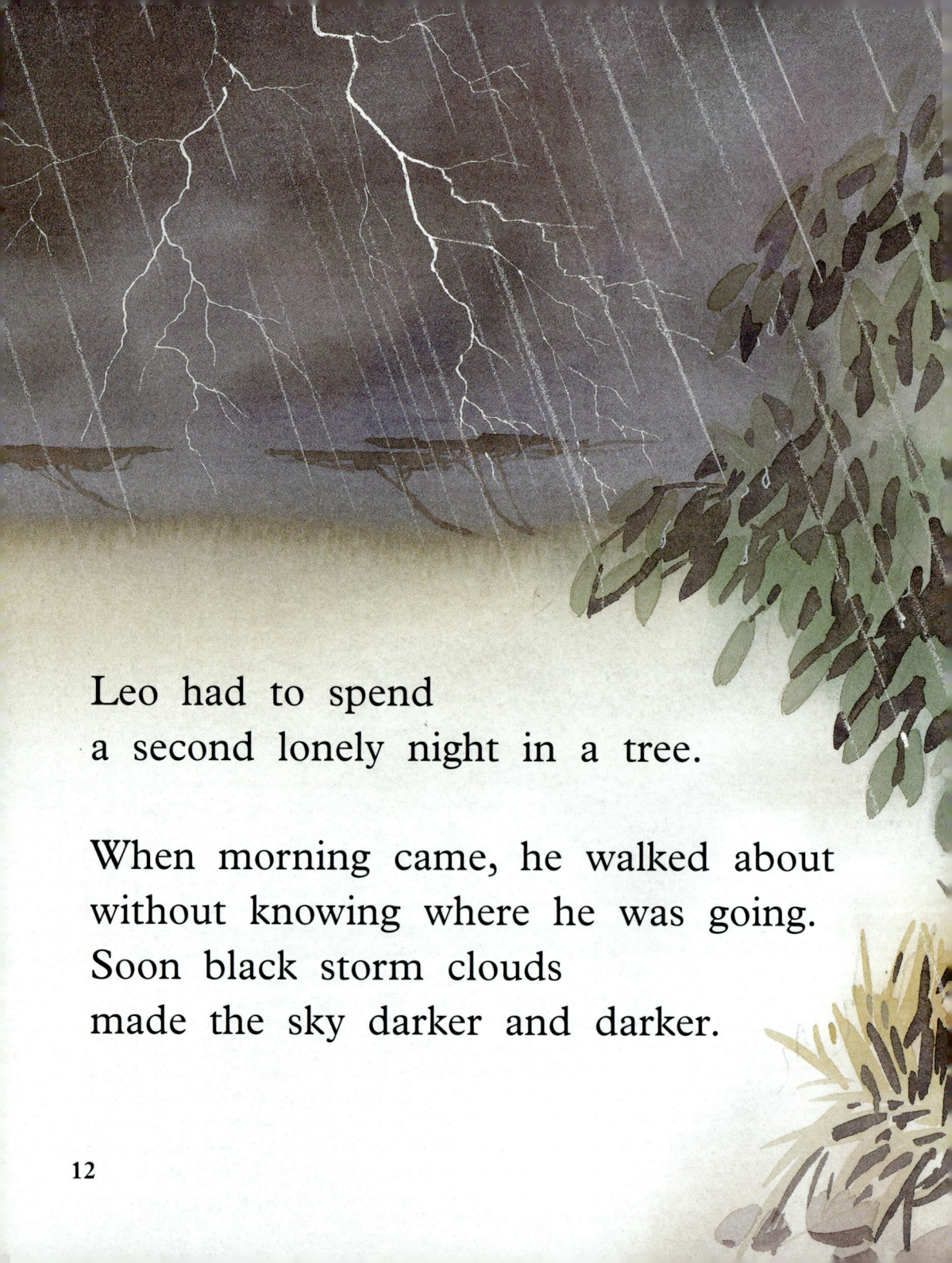

When morning came, he walked about
without knowing where he was going.
Soon black storm clouds
made the sky darker and darker.

Then lightning flashed
and thunder roared.
Heavy rain came pouring down.
The storm went on for hours.

Leo crouched under a low bush all night,
but he could not keep dry.

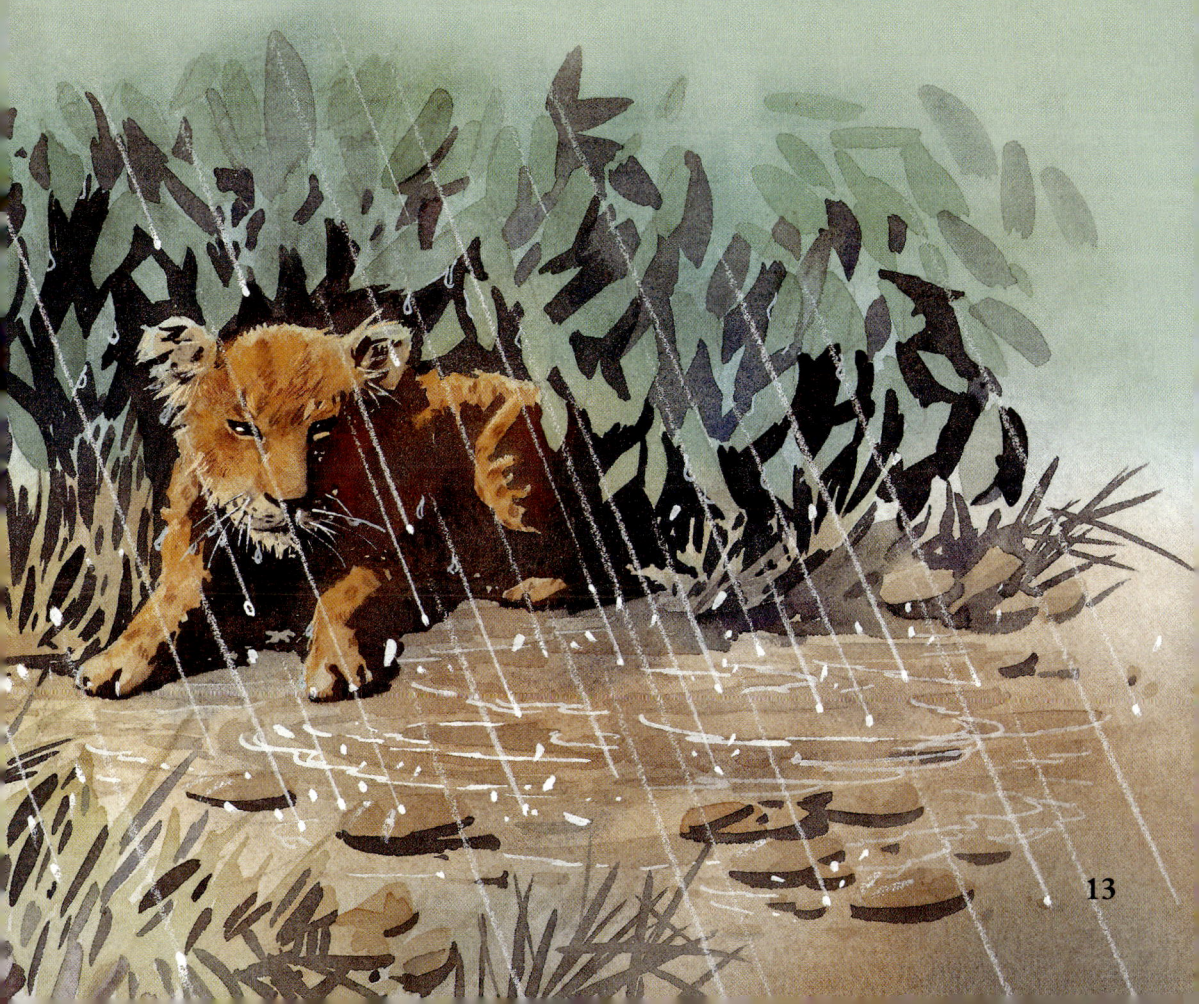

The next morning,
Leo looked half-drowned.

He was too young to hunt for food.
It had been three days
since his last meal.
If he did not find his family soon,
he would die.

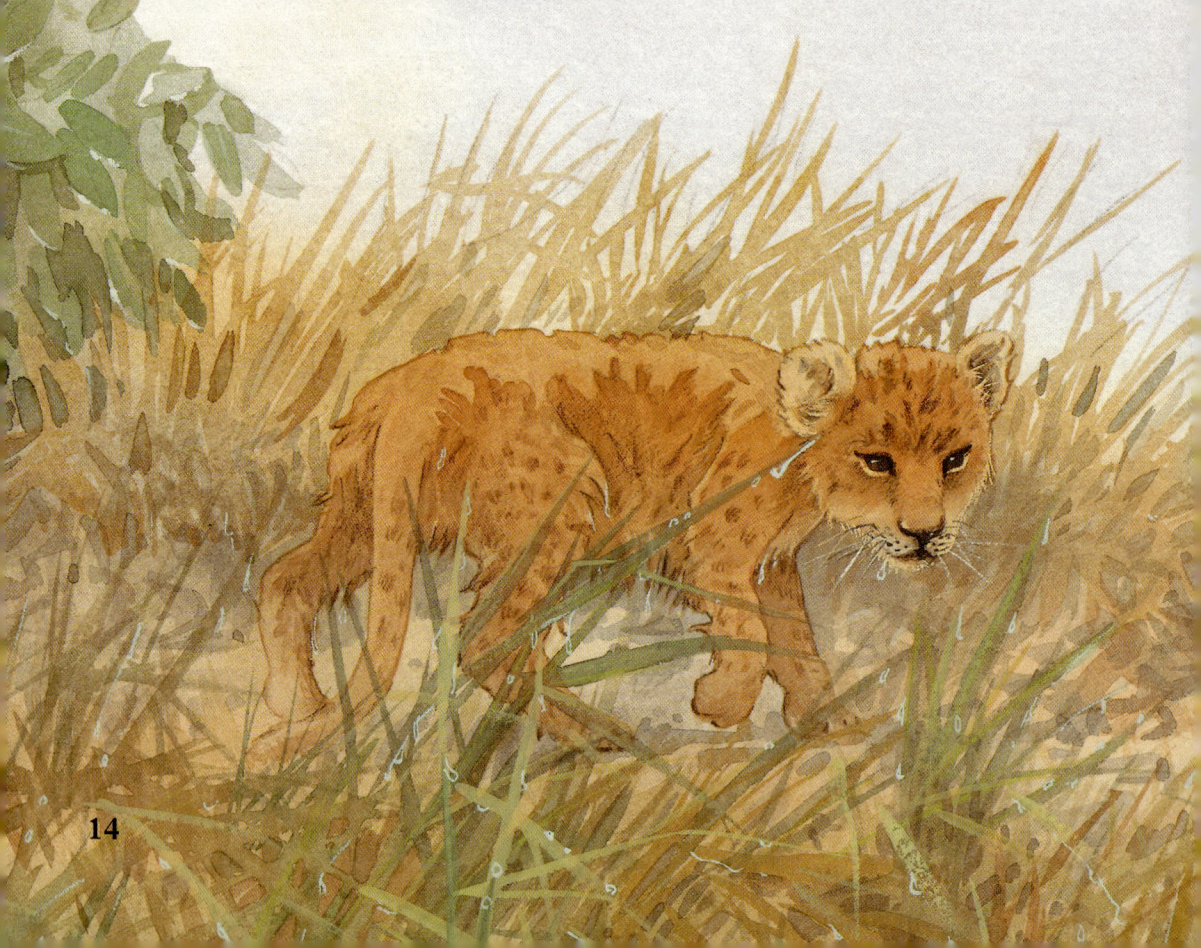

Suddenly, Leo heard a lion
roaring in the distance.
He knew that roar!
Now he knew where the pride was,
and he set off again.

Leo struggled on through the wet grass.
He was very tired,
but he was not going to give up now!

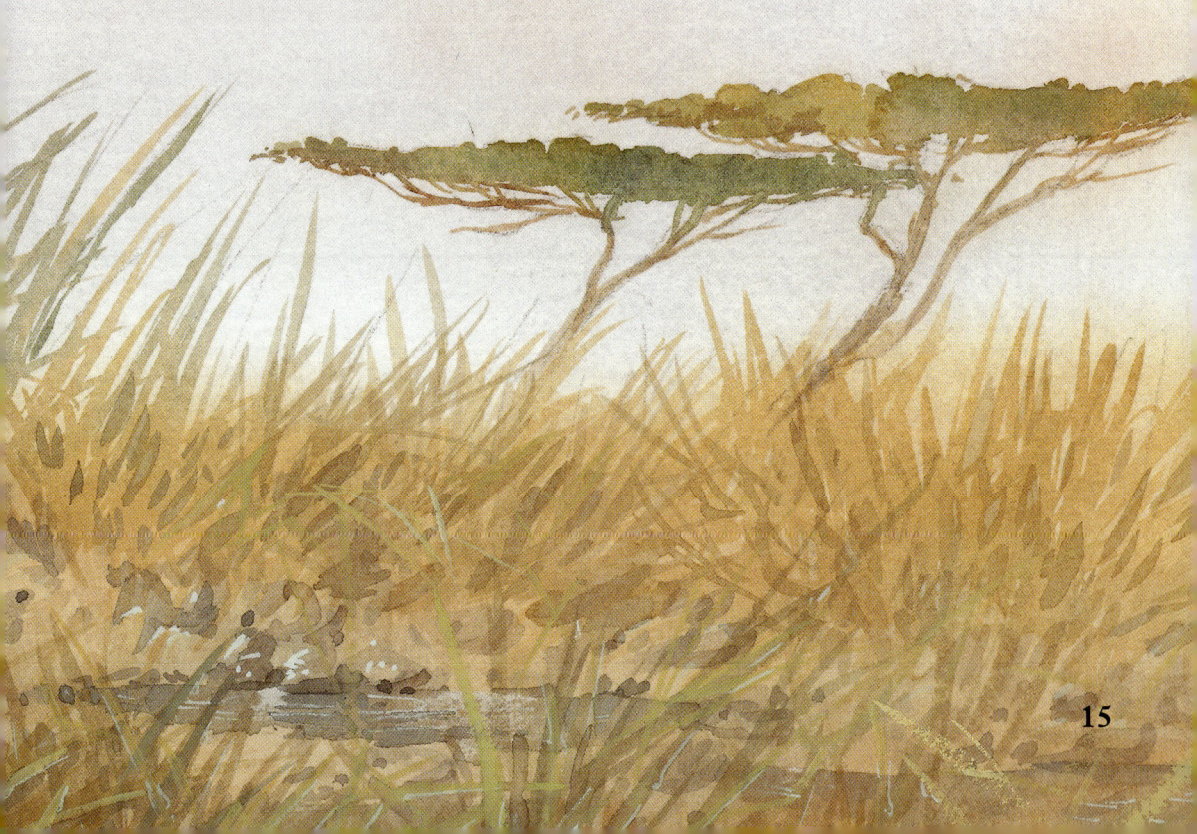

And, at last,
Leo reached his family.
He was so glad to find them!
His aunts licked him all over
and fed him.

Then he lay down beside them
and slept... and slept... and slept.

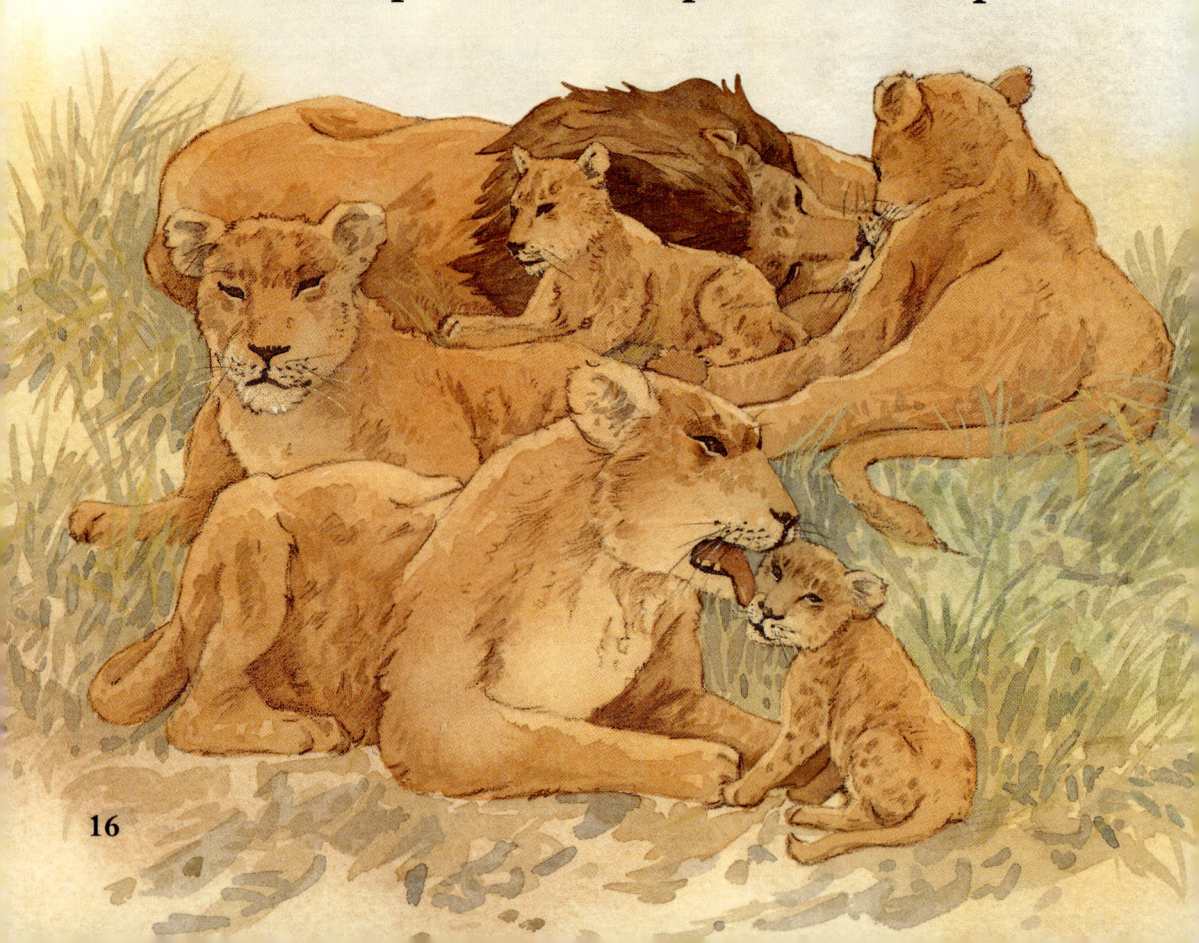